MASTERING CHRONIC PAIN
A Professional's Guide to Behavioral Treatment

Robert N. Jamison, PhD

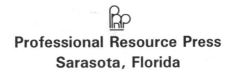

Professional Resource Press
Sarasota, Florida

Published by Professional Resource Press
(An imprint of Professional Resource Exchange, Inc.)
Post Office Box 15560
Sarasota, FL 34277-1560

The copy editor for this book was David Anson, the managing editor was Debbie Fink, the production coordinator was Laurie Girsch, and the cover was created by Jami's Graphic Design.

Library of Congress Cataloging-in-Publication Data

Jamison, Robert N. date.
    Mastering chronic pain : a professional's guide to behavioral treatment / Robert N. Jamison.
        p.   cm.
    Companion v. to: Learning to Master Your Chronic Pain.
    Includes bibliographical references.
    ISBN 1-56887-018-3 (pbk. : alk. paper)
    1. Chronic pain--Treatment. 2. Cognitive therapy. 3. Behavior therapy.   I. Title.
    [DNLM: 1. Pain--therapy. 2. Chronic Disease--therapy.
3. Cognitive Therapy.   WL 704 J32m 1996]
RB127.J253 1996
616'.0472--dc20
DNLM/DLC
for Library of Congress   96-16713
                                            CIP

DEDICATION

This book is dedicated to my parents,
Ruth and Wallace Jamison,
with love and gratitude.

TABLE OF CONTENTS

CHAPTER 4 *(Continued)*

PREFACE

This therapist's manual was written to accompany the patient's handbook, *Learning to Master Your Chronic Pain* (Jamison, 1996b). It is designed to assist therapists in organizing and implementing a structured, time-limited pain program. It describes a program that is built on sound psychological principles of cognitive/behavioral therapy and rehabilitation. This book, along with the patient's handbook, will assist a clinician in organizing a structured pain management program for persons referred for treatment of chronic pain. This program may be hospital or university based or may stand alone. Participants may be patients whose persistent nonmalignant pain has been treated with little success. Many of the patients referred to a pain management program have seen several specialists, had many diagnostic tests, and undergone repeated physical therapy, nerve blocks, chiropractic treatment, surgery, and psychotherapy. In most cases the pain has lasted for years, with minimal long-term benefit from treatment. This text details an alternative approach to the management of chronic pain.

The program outlined is designed to be part of a multidisciplinary pain center. Patients participating in a structured pain program should be under the care of a physician and have access to medical treatment. A therapist who runs a pain program should have experience in the diagnosis and treatment of persons with chronic pain. The therapist may have graduate and postgraduate training in psychology and behavioral medicine or extensive therapy experience with chronic pain patients. A number of other specialists (including psychologists, psychiatrists, social workers, nurses, and medical practitioners) who have indirect involvement in a pain management program may also benefit from this book.

This program is designed to be flexible in meeting the individual needs of the persons served. The handbook is structured much like a course text. The facilitator is encouraged to choose specific topics that are most appropriate for the individuals and the group. The participants are assigned homework and encouraged to complete the checklists and questionnaires. The more ways that the patient can participate in the program the greater the likelihood that the information will be remembered and used. The program may consist of multiple sessions throughout the day or weekly sessions for a series of weeks. The facilitator should experiment with different group formats and techniques in order to best meet the needs of the patients. Groups consisting of six to eight members are optimal, but larger and smaller groups are also workable. Furthermore, the handbook for patients may be used in individual sessions.

Included in the therapist's guide is a description of components of the program, the roles of a team, program goals, patient selection criteria, and information on program evaluation. Much of the information in the guide is derived from published studies and clinical research. Professionals such as general practitioners, medical specialists, nurses, physical therapists, vocational rehabilitation counselors, pastoral counselors, exercise physiologists, and occupational therapists may find this book to be a useful resource.

The ultimate goal of any program for persons with chronic pain is to relieve suffering and alleviate a persistent, stressful condition. Both the patient's handbook and the therapist's guide were written because of the effectiveness of pain management techniques in improving the quality of life for individuals experiencing pain. Patient helpfulness ratings after treatment and at follow-up have demonstrated the benefits of these approaches. The usefulness of behavioral medicine strategies is now undisputed, and these strategies are seen as an important component of treatment for chronic pain. Future investigations should determine which characteristics of patients predict benefit from a cognitive/behavioral treatment approach and which treatment strategies are cost-effective and of greatest use in combating an epidemic of disability due to chronic pain. These books offer a structure in which outcome can be assessed. The author encourages collaborative investigations of the best ways to treat individuals experiencing daily pain.

The production of this therapist's guide and the patient handbook could not have been possible without the help and encouragement of the many patients and colleagues with whom I have worked over the years. I am indebted to those patients who taught me the ways they cope with suffering and pain. I acknowledge with thanks the staff at the Pain Management Center of Brigham and Women's Hospital. I especially wish to thank Julie McCoy and Jaylyn Olivo for their editorial assistance.* Finally, I am most grateful to my wife, Lisa, for her support and understanding, and to our two children, Mary and Paul, for their tolerance during those hours I was away completing these books.

---

*The material used in this text was adapted from many sources. Every effort was made to acknowledge these sources. I apologize for any unintended omissions which may have occurred.

MASTERING CHRONIC PAIN
A Professional's Guide to
Behavioral Treatment

CHAPTER 1

Theoretical Issues
of Chronic Pain

Scott* was in good health before he sustained a work-related injury a year and a half ago, when he fell from a scaffold at a construction site. Since the fall he has complained of low back pain and pain radiating down his right leg. MRI and CT showed evidence of a marginal disc bulge. However, Scott was not considered a candidate for surgery. He was evaluated by many physicians, including his own doctor, an orthopedic surgeon, a neurologist, and a neurosurgeon. Many different kinds of medication were prescribed. Scott was seen by a physical therapist twice a week for 6 months and received regular ultrasound and heat-pack treatments. Still he showed little improvement.

Over the past year Scott gained weight and developed poor posture. His leg and abdominal muscles became weak. He was assessed by a psychiatrist, who determined that he was depressed, anxious, angry, and potentially suicidal. Because of being out of work and being inactive, he had financial worries and ongoing family conflicts. Scott could not sleep at night and instead napped during the day. He no longer shared a bed with his wife because his inability to sleep kept her up most of the night. They no longer made love because this increased his pain. Scott became severely depressed and irritable. He had problems concentrating and remembering things, and he felt frustrated because he could not complete even simple tasks. He became increasingly hopeless about his condition.

Scott's story is much like those of millions of other people who have been devastated by ongoing pain. Chronic nonmalignant pain is a costly syndrome that influences every aspect of a person's functioning. Profound changes in quality of life are associated with intractable chronic pain. Significant interference with sleep, employment, social functioning, and daily activities is common. Chronic pain patients frequently report

---

*Names and identifying information have been disguised throughout this book to protect patient confidentiality.

depression, anxiety, irritability, sexual dysfunction, and decreased energy. Family roles are altered, and worries about financial limitations and future consequences of a restricted lifestyle abound. Chronic pain patients generally present with a history of multiple medical procedures yielding minimal physical findings. The treatments used for acute pain are often insufficient or inappropriate for chronic pain. The cycle of pain and depression is illustrated in Figure 1.1 (below).

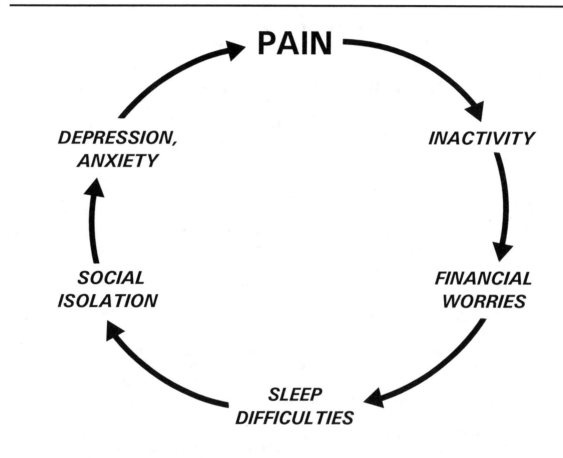

Figure 1.1. Pain Cycle.

The statistics on chronic pain are staggering. Dr. John Bonica, a founding member of the American Pain Society, estimated that chronic pain syndromes afflict a third of the American population, or more than 80 million people (Bonica, 1992). Pain is the major reason for visiting a primary care physician, and more than 50 million people are temporarily disabled by pain. More than 550 million work days were lost in 1989 because of chronic pain. This figure translates into a current cost of more than $85 billion a year in lost productivity, lost wages, workers' compensation, and medical expenses. Drs. John Frymoyer and William Cats-Baril reviewed the literature and compiled further statistics on the impact of chronic low back pain in America and concluded that the total costs of low back disorders could be inflated into the $75 to $100 billion range (Frymoyer & Cats-Baril, 1991). Seventy million see a physician each year for pain and 4 billion work days are lost due to pain. The *Nuprin Pain Report* - a survey of individuals across the United States - confirmed in 1985 that 15% of the general population (26 million people) suffered from back pain for more than 30 consecutive days sometime in their career (*Nuprin Pain Report*, 1985). Seventy-three percent of those surveyed reported at least one headache, 56% experienced backaches, 53% had muscle pain, and 51% reported joint pains. Pain described as the "most troublesome" included backaches (16%), headaches (15%), joint pains (11%), stomach pains (6%), muscle pains (5%), premenstrual and menstrual pains (3%), and dental pains (3%). More than 14% of all Americans missed at least 1 day of work per year because of pain.

PAIN CATEGORIES

Just as there are many different kinds of pain, there are a number of ways to categorize pain according to the character and history of the symptom. *Acute pain* is self-limiting, is usually of less than 6 months' duration, and is generally adaptive in nature; examples are postsurgical pain, dental pain, and pain following an injury. *Chronic non-malignant pain* persists beyond 6 months and is intractable. Pain severity may vary with no known relation to active pathophysiologic or pathoanatomic processes; examples are chronic mechanical low back pain and diffuse myofascial pain. *Recurrent acute pain* consists of a series of intermittent episodes of pain that are acute in character but chronic insofar as the condition persists for more than 6 months (e.g., migraine headaches, trigeminal neuralgia, and temporomandibular disorder). *Chronic progressive pain* increases in severity over time and often is associated with malignancies and degenerative disorders such as skeletal metastatic disease and rheumatoid arthritis.

Acute pain is generally associated with tissue damage and represents a warning of injury to the individual. It is expected to be directly proportional to the nociceptive sensory input induced by the tissue damage and to continue until the damaged tissue and/or afferent pathways have returned to normal functioning. Chronic pain, in contrast, is a persistent condition often associated with an initial episode of acute pain but continuing long past the time when healing would normally take place. Chronic pain serves no beneficial purpose and is resistant to medical intervention.

It is popularly recognized that chronic pain is a multifaceted phenomenon which includes the dimensions of nociception, perception, appraisal, behavior, and social environmental influences. Because nociception is a private experience, what can be learned about how pain is being experienced depends on what the patient says and does. The International Association for the Study of Pain (IASP) defines pain as what each individual says it is. An IASP subcommittee chaired by Dr. Harold Mersky developed a list of terms commonly used in describing the experience of pain. The abbreviated definitions are presented in Table 1.1 (below).

TABLE 1.1: COMMONLY USED TERMS FOR PAIN

Pain Terms	Abbreviated Definition
Allodynia	Pain resulting from a nonnoxious stimulus to normal skin
Analgesia	Absence of pain on noxious stimulation
Anesthesia dolorosa	Pain in an area or region that is anesthetic
Causalgia	Sustained burning pain after a traumatic nerve lesion
Central pain	Associated with a lesion of the Central Nervous System (CNS)
Dysesthesia	An unpleasant abnormal sensation
Hyperalgesia	Increased sensitivity to noxious stimulation
Hyperesthesia	Increased sensitivity to stimulation
Hyperpathia	A painful syndrome characterized by overreaction and aftersensation to stimuli
Hypoalgesia	Diminished sensitivity to noxious stimulation
Neuralgia	Pain in the distribution of the nerve
Neuritis	Inflammation of a nerve
Neuropathy	Disturbance in the function of or pathological change in a nerve
Nociceptor	A receptor preferentially sensitive to a noxious or potentially noxious stimulus
Noxious	Tissue-damaging
Pain	An unpleasant sensory and emotional experience associated with actual or potential tissue damage or described in terms of such damage
Pain threshold	The least stimulus intensity at which a subject perceives pain
Pain tolerance level	The greatest stimulus intensity causing pain that a subject is prepared to tolerate

---

PSYCHOGENIC VERSUS ORGANIC PAIN

Chronic pain represents a complex interaction of factors. The pain may be related to an initial somatic event but, over time, may be increasingly influenced by the patient's personality, beliefs, and environment. Attempts to distinguish reliably between organic and psychogenic pain have been largely unsuccessful. Some practitioners incorrectly believe that chronic pain reflects either organic pathology or psychogenic symptoms. If physical findings are inadequate to account for a patient's report of chronic pain, then the pain is perceived to be largely psychological. It is generally unwarranted to assume that psychological factors are the primary cause of pain. Whether an individual presents with clear evidence of organic pathology may be independent of whether there is significant psychopathology. For example, a person may have both a major psychiatric illness and clinical low back pain. Until ways are developed to detect and quantify pain objectively, we must believe that pain exists when the patient says it does, and we must recognize that it is not valid to diagnose pain as a purely psychological phenomenon.

MODELS FOR
TREATING CHRONIC PAIN

A number of treatment models directly influence how chronic pain is diagnosed and treated. The most traditional is the *biomedical model*, in which symptoms are considered to represent underlying disease. Management consists of a correct diagnosis and treatment aimed at resolving the problem. Various interventions for pain are tried until the best approach is found.

In the *psychiatric model*, pain is influenced by conscious and unconscious psychiatric processes. The aim of therapy is to identify unconscious conflicts and unmet emotional needs, with the ultimate goal of diminishing pain by resolving these problems. This model fits well with the biomedical model. If pain persists after all medical interventions have been tried, psychological factors are suspected as the primary determinant of pain. In both the biomedical and the psychiatric models, the interventions offered are intended to treat the underlying cause of pain.

In the *behavioral model*, pain is believed to be influenced most by consequences in the environment. The goal of treatment is to change environmental cues and learned behaviors in order to maximize functional capacity and minimize perception of pain and distress. In other words, this model assumes that a restructuring of the patient's environment is needed in order to change behaviors and perceptions.

Unfortunately, none of these three models is effective in and of itself in resolving chronic pain.

All of these models have now been combined into the *biopsychosocial model*. In this model, chronic pain is considered to be influenced by medical, psychiatric, behavioral, and personality factors. Thus emphasis is placed on a multidisciplinary approach to treatment that encompasses medical interventions, insight therapy, education, and behavioral therapy - in other words, elements designed to address all dimensions of the pain experience. Efforts are made to change the patient's perception of the problem and to revise the patient's expectations, focusing on relief rather than cure and on slow improvement rather than immediate resolution. Patients are encouraged to participate actively in their treatment in order to decrease their pain, reduce the degree of their disability, improve their emotional functioning, and decrease their reliance on the health care system. The ultimate goal is to gain control over the pain.

UNIMODAL
TREATMENT APPROACHES

The many ways to treat chronic pain include medication, manipulation, injections, acupuncture, ultrasound, hot packs, transcutaneous electrical nerve stimulation, psychotherapy, and surgery. Traditionally, these modalities would be tried one at a time in the hope that one approach would eventually work. Although most individuals with acute pain benefit, many patients with chronic pain do not, and in some cases a pattern of failure and disability develops.

When a particular treatment fails to eradicate the pain, the patient is often sent to another health care professional, who may institute some other therapy. This cycle of treatment by many clinicians with many individual therapies can result in multiple evaluations, medications, and hospitalizations and can lead to increased depression, dependence, and deconditioning.

An alternative strategy for chronic pain patients is a structured, goal-oriented program in which professionals from different disciplines work together to manage the pain with the patient's active participation.

> Scott's story is a successful one. When referred to a pain management program by his general practitioner, Scott identified his goals. He stated that he wanted to (a) increase his physical endurance so that he could stand and sit for up to 2 hours; (b) socialize with friends on a regular basis and engage in some recreational activities; (c) learn ways to pace his activity; (d) eat out once a week and attend his son's sporting events; (e) improve his mood and prevent future depressive episodes; and (f) learn about opportunities for retraining so that he could return to work on a part-time or full-time basis.
>
> Scott attended a 10-week, group-based outpatient pain program. He rated his pain on a daily basis and noted decreasing pain scores. Despite discomfort, he established a daily exercise regimen and gradually increased his endurance, standing and sitting for longer periods. Scott increased the duration of his cardiovascular exercises from 10 minutes to 1 hour each day. He used a treadmill at the program and reported walking on a regular basis at home.
>
> Scott was able to use medication responsibly. He decreased his intake of tranquilizing and narcotic medication. His goal was not to rely on any prescription medication for the relief of his pain. Scott actively participated in group discussions and pain management classes. He benefited from interacting with other group members. He remained positive and optimistic about the management of his pain, exhibiting minimal pain behavior and complaining little. Scott benefited from educational and cognitive/behavioral therapy and had an improved sense of well-being at the conclusion of the program.

Scott's participation in the pain program dramatically affected his beliefs about his ability to cope. He learned that he could successfully participate in activities despite discomfort. He became more confident that through pain management strategies he could indeed reduce his pain. He learned to keep pain from interfering with his sleep and to cope with mild to moderate pain. He maintained his home exercise program (walking and using a stationary bike). He came to perceive himself as having more control over his pain.

Six months after completing the pain program, Scott was still walking three times a week and was engaging in weight-training exercises every other day. He regularly used relaxation strategies, self-hypnosis, and distraction techniques. At this point, he met with a vocational rehabilitation counselor and took a functional-capacity screening test. Following an evaluation of his vocational opportunities, he began training as a foreman and as an inspector of construction sites. Scott eventually returned to his former place of employment. In general, Scott appeared to be coping well and managing his pain with less anxiety, depression, and irritability.

CHAPTER 2

Program Description

RATIONALE FOR A
GROUP-BASED PROGRAM

This section presents an overview of psychological and behavioral interventions for chronic noncancer pain in the context of a multidisciplinary pain management program. The topics reviewed include the rationale for a group-based program, the program goals, the roles played by members of a multidisciplinary team, and program components and evaluation.

A group-based pain management program offers some distinct advantages over individual unimodal treatment. First, most pain patients have similar needs. Thus, information can be presented more efficiently to a group than to individuals. Second, group processes can help change behavior. Patients seem to benefit from interacting with other people with chronic pain. Group members can encourage each other to practice relaxation, exercise regularly, and maintain a positive attitude. Third, a structured time-limited program offers definite goals, rules, and end points. Patients know what they can realistically expect and are given clear feedback regarding their participation in the program's activities.

Fourth, pain management programs are cost-effective. Patients who complete a multidisciplinary pain program return to work or undergo vocational rehabilitation more often than patients who do not enter a pain program. Such programs also produce marked subjective and functional improvements: pain ratings decrease from admission to discharge, reliance on medication decreases, and physical functioning increases. These positive outcomes have been shown to be maintained 2 to 3 years after completion of the program.

Finally, pain management programs offer comprehensive assessments and discharge plans. Because of the multifaceted, structured nature of a group-based program, a comprehensive treatment evaluation is easily attainable. A multidisciplinary staff can design a discharge and follow-up plan to meet the needs of each patient.

Interdisciplinary pain management programs have been shown to be more effective than unimodal approaches.   Flor, Fydrich, and Turk (1992), in a meta-analysis of outcome data from 65 studies, found that (a) combined treatments are superior to single treatments or no treatments for chronic nonmalignant pain; (b) participation in an interdisciplinary pain program increases the return-to-work rate (average, 43%) and decreases health care utilization; (c) the benefits of an interdisciplinary pain program are maintained over time; and (d) patients who benefit from treatment and those who do not are similar in terms of age, pain duration, workers' compensation status, and treatment duration.

GOALS OF THE PROGRAM

At the start of a program, each patient should identify specific goals. These may include the following:

1. *Reduction of Pain Intensity.* Although patients rarely if ever report that their pain has been eliminated, by the conclusion of the program they often report a reduction in the amount of pain. Most patients enter a pain management program because of persistent pain, but they are taught not to set pain elimination as their primary goal. Instead they are encouraged to focus on other, more attainable goals.
2. *Enhancement of Physical Functioning.* In group-based pain programs, patients are encouraged to participate regularly in exercise (including stretching, cardiovascular reconditioning, and weight training) and to increase their activity at a progressive rate under supervision. The goal is to gradually increase function without exceeding predetermined limits of pain and discomfort. Patients have been known to increase their physical strength and endurance by 50% to 100% over a 3-month period.
3. *Proper Use of Medication.* Through education and daily monitoring, most patients are able to use prescription pain medication responsibly. Participants are frequently asked to monitor their medication for a week before entering a program and to report their daily medication at the end of the program.
4. *Improvement of Sleep, Mood, and Interaction With Other People.* Most patients report being depressed and having problems relating to other people. At the conclusion of most group-based pain programs, patients usually show evidence of improved sleep, decreased emotional distress, and increased self-esteem.

5. *Return to Work or to Normal Daily Activities.* Patients who set as their goal an eventual return to work are often successful. Follow-up helpfulness ratings indicate that patients who have a positive experience in a pain management program tend to return to work and/or maintain an active, productive lifestyle.

ROLES OF A
MULTIDISCIPLINARY TEAM

Chronic pain involves a complex interaction of physiological and psychosocial factors, and successful intervention requires the coordinated effort of a treatment team with expertise in a variety of therapeutic disciplines. Although some pain centers offer a unimodal treatment approach, most programs use a blend of medical, psychological, vocational, and educational techniques. Generally included are medical assessment, medication management, pain-reduction treatments, didactic instruction, relaxation training, biofeedback, physical therapy, psychotherapy, and vocational counseling.

Most interdisciplinary pain treatment programs have as their core staff one or more physicians, a clinical psychologist, and a physical therapist. Other health professionals who may play important roles include clinical nurse specialists, occupational therapists, vocational rehabilitation counselors, and exercise physiologists. Physicians from specialty areas (e.g., neurology, rheumatology, orthopedic surgery, physical medicine, internal medicine) should be available for consultation. The physician's primary responsibility is to oversee the medical aspects of treatment and to prescribe medication and procedures when needed. The psychologist, psychiatrist, or social worker addresses the mental health and behavioral aspects of the patient's program. He or she may facilitate the pain management classes and group therapy sessions and may offer training in biofeedback and relaxation. The physical therapist and exercise physiologist coordinate daily group exercises and assist patients in setting up and following individual exercise programs. An interdisciplinary staff coordinates efforts to rehabilitate the patient and designs a comprehensive discharge and follow-up plan to meet each patient's short- and long-term needs. The patient's participation is strongly encouraged. Among the predictors of success in a multidisciplinary pain program are the patient's motivation to cope with pain and the patient's support system outside the program.

PROGRAM STRUCTURE

Multidisciplinary pain programs are often highly structured, time limited, and organized along a specific treatment schedule. Common goals include an increase in physical, social, and emotional functioning and a decrease in pain and in reliance on health care services. The patient is expected to attend clinic sessions and to participate in all aspects of the program. These expectations must be made clear. To this end, patients frequently sign a treatment contract that spells out the general program requirements as well as individual treatment goals. An example of a treatment contract is presented on pages 13 and 14. In addition to helping patients understand exactly what is expected of them, such a contract is a means of identifying before treatment those patients who may lack motivation or have difficulty conforming to the structure of the program. Patients are asked to keep a daily written record of their pain intensity, medication use, and activity levels. Noncompliance may be grounds for discharge from the program.

Table 2.1 (below) lists some treatment modalities commonly used for chronic pain patients participating in a pain management program.

TABLE 2.1: TREATMENT MODALITIES FOR CHRONIC PAIN

---

1. Medical assessment
2. Psychological evaluation and testing
3. Medication
4. Nerve blocks, trigger point therapy
5. Relaxation training
6. Biofeedback
7. Physical therapy
8. Transcutaneous Electrical Nerve Stimulation (TENS)
9. Acupuncture
10. Nutrition counseling
11. Occupational therapy
12. Education: group and individual instruction
13. Support groups
14. Psychotherapy
15. Vocational counseling
16. Surgery and implantable devices

SAMPLE PATIENT CONTRACT*

The purpose of this agreement is for me, Ms. Rea L. Paine, to understand and agree with Dr. Robert Jamison, (representing the treatment team), and Mr. Noel Paine (a member of my family or someone else who is significant to me) on the following:

1. The Pain Management Program is designed to help me learn to cope with my pain. The goals include changing those actions and attitudes that are associated with the pain and learning to manage my life in ways that will be more satisfying.
2. An overall goal is to gain control of my pain so that I can do more things that are considered normal for a person my age. Specifically, I have the following goals:

    a. I will work to decrease my pain by 25% by using techniques described in the course.
    b. I will use my medication appropriately on a regularly scheduled basis and work to decrease my use of prescription medication.
    c. I will engage in a regular exercise program consisting of swimming three times a week and walking every day.
    d. I will learn ways to improve my mood so that I will be less depressed and anxious.
    e. I will go out to eat and go to a movie with my family twice a month.
    f. I will have a definite vocational plan and enter a retraining program

3. I agree to become less reliant on pain medications as I increase my activity level. I agree to record all medications that I am presently taking for 1 week at the start of the program and for 1 week before the end of the program.
4. I will keep records showing my progress. I understand that I am responsible for these records. I will keep my records up to date and available for inspection.
5. I recognize that members of my family and others significant to me are considered essential in helping me to break old habits and to learn new ways to live with my pain. As a result, I will actively encourage these individuals to participate in my program. In addition, I understand that you may talk with me or with members of my family if that will improve the chances of my attaining my goals. I understand that I will be informed before other people are contacted.
6. I understand that I am expected to attend all scheduled sessions and to participate in all at-home activities. *Pain is no excuse.* I further understand that my absence for a total of 3 days will be grounds for dropping me from the program.
7. I will immediately inform the staff about other medical appointments, changes in treatment, or changes in medications.
8. On the basis of my treatment needs, members of the treatment team will decide what the follow-up components of the program will be and how long follow-up will continue.

I understand and agree to the above conditions, and I acknowledge that the Pain Management Program at Brigham and Women's Hospital has now been explained to my satisfaction.

_____   _____
(Patient)   (Date)
_____   _____
(Team Representative)   (Date)
_____   _____
(Significant Other)   (Date)

*Note: Adapted from "Behavioral Treatment of Chronic Pain," by M. J. Follick, D. K. Ahern, and E. W. Aberger, in *Applications in Behavioral Medicine and Health Psychology: A Clinicians Source Book* (pp. 266-267), by J. A. Blumenthal and D. C. McKee (Eds.), 1987, Sarasota, FL: Professional Resource Exchange. Copyright © 1987 by Professional Resource Exchange, Inc. Adapted with permission.

PATIENT CONTRACT

The purpose of this agreement is for me, _____, to understand and agree with _____, (representing the treatment team), and _____ (a member of my family or someone else who is significant to me) on the following:

1. The Pain Management Program is designed to help me learn to cope with my pain. The goals include changing those actions and attitudes that are associated with the pain and learning to manage my life in ways that will be more satisfying.
2. An overall goal is to gain control of my pain so that I can do more things that are considered normal for a person my age. Specifically, I have the following goals:

   a. _____
   b. _____
   c. _____
   d. _____
   e. _____
   f. _____

3. I agree to become less reliant on pain medications as I increase my activity level. I agree to record all medications that I am presently taking for 1 week at the start of the program and for 1 week before the end of the program.
4. I will keep records showing my progress. I understand that I am responsible for these records. I will keep my records up to date and available for inspection.
5. I recognize that members of my family and others significant to me are considered essential in helping me to break old habits and to learn new ways to live with my pain. As a result, I will actively encourage these individuals to participate in my program. In addition, I understand that you may talk with me or with members of my family if that will improve the chances of my attaining my goals. I understand that I will be informed before other people are contacted.
6. I understand that I am expected to attend all scheduled sessions and to participate in all at-home activities. *Pain is no excuse.* I further understand that my absence for a total of 3 days will be grounds for dropping me from the program.
7. I will immediately inform the staff about other medical appointments, changes in treatment, or changes in medications.
8. On the basis of my treatment needs, members of the treatment team will decide what the follow-up components of the program will be and how long follow-up will continue.

I understand and agree to the above conditions, and I acknowledge that the Pain Management Program at _____ has now been explained to my satisfaction.

_____   _____
(Patient)   (Date)

_____   _____
(Team Representative)   (Date)

_____   _____
(Significant Other)   (Date)

CHAPTER 3

Assessment and Patient Selection Issues

MEDICAL ASSESSMENT OF CHRONIC PAIN

Before a patient is admitted into a structured outpatient program for chronic pain, all of his or her medical evaluations must be reviewed. Patients should be referred to the program by a physician. The referral letter should include a detailed pain history, results of a comprehensive physical examination, a neurologic and musculoskeletal assessment, laboratory and radiologic findings, and a diagnosis. Information about pain onset and a description of the current condition (e.g., location, distribution, quality, severity, and duration) should be included as well. It may be necessary to request copies of clinical notes or to call the referring physician to establish whether the pain represents anything other than a chronic nonmalignant condition.

The physical examination should rule out any underlying progressive disease. The patient's general physical, neurologic, and musculoskeletal findings and mental health status should be evaluated. Information obtained at general physical examination should include response to palpation, motion, heat, and cold; body posture; aggravating factors; and range of motion. The neurologic examination should include an assessment of cranial function, sympathetic function, and cerebral function and tests of spinal nerves. The musculoskeletal examination should include an evaluation of neck, upper extremity, trunk, and lower extremity muscles. Results of radiographic procedures such as magnetic resonance imaging (MRI), computed tomography (CT), and electromyography (EMG) should be reviewed. Patients who have unresolved medical issues may need clearance to participate in the exercise component of the program. Patients with a history of cancer or a diagnosis of spinal stenosis, acute osteomyelitis, acute herniated disk, or any clinically unstable systemic illness may require additional information from the referring physician before being accepted into a structured pain program. An example of a physician's medical evaluation form is presented on pages 29-32. Detailed information on the medical evaluation of a chronic pain patient can be obtained elsewhere (Bonica & Loeser, 1990; Erickson, 1989; Raj, 1992).

Unfortunately, considerable subjectivity is inherent in the physical examination of a chronic pain patient. The concordance of examination findings among clinicians is often low, as is agreement about an organic versus nonorganic source of pain. Reviews by Drs. Gorden Waddell (1982), Dennis Turk and Ronald Melzack (1992), and Sridhar Vasudevan (1992) conclude that there is no direct relationship among pain, its pathology, and functional impairment. Dr. Gordon Waddell (1982) proposed that back pain can be separated into three broad groups: (a) mechanical pain (pain related to physical activity); (b) neuropathic pain (nerve root pain), and (c) pain due to serious pathology. He identified nine indicators for serious spinal pathology: (a) an age less than 20 or more than 55 years; (b) pain in the midback area (rather than the neck or low back); (c) pain unrelated to physical activity or duration of activity; (d) a history of cancer; (e) total-body symptoms, such as dramatic weight loss; (f) limited movement of the spine; (g) major back deformity; (h) an elevated erythrocyte sedimentation rate; and (i) abnormal x-ray results. If any suspicions arise that a participant has an undiagnosed illness, he or she should be referred back to the primary physician.

PSYCHOLOGICAL ASSESSMENT

It is more important to know what kind of a person has a disease
than what kind of a disease a person has.

Sir William Osler

It can safely be argued that the sensation of pain is a personal experience that cannot be measured objectively. Because pain is a subjective state, its measurement relies both on what the patient says and on what the patient does in response to the pain. A number of psychosocial factors contribute to pain: attitudes, beliefs, cultural norms, moods, focus of attention, motivation, and personality traits. For example, individuals who take a placebo that they believe is a strong pain reliever report significant decreases in pain intensity. Persons who are anxious or depressed tend to report more intense pain than those who are experiencing minimal emotional distress. Persons with pain who are distracted by other matters report less pain intensity.   Further, certain personality traits may tend to predispose individuals toward greater tolerance of pain (e.g., emotionally stable extroverts tolerate pain better than anxious introverts).

The process of initially assessing the chronic pain patient is much like piecing together parts of a puzzle. The collected information must then be used to determine a prognosis and the best course of treatment. Important components that must be evaluated in this process include pain intensity, functional capacity, mood and personality, active or passive coping (e.g., distracting oneself rather than dwelling on the pain), and medication usage. In addition, a behavioral analysis should be conducted, and information on psychosocial history, adverse effects of treatment, and health care utilization should be obtained. Subsequent sections will highlight ways to assess each of these areas and will discuss some of the strengths and weaknesses of the assessment process.

USEFULNESS OF PSYCHOMETRIC MEASURES

Standardized psychometric testing methods are frequently used to evaluate the psychological functioning of chronic pain patients. Unfortunately, most traditional testing tools were designed to evaluate psychopathology in persons with significant mental dysfunction. Although most chronic pain patients state that they are depressed and anxious, seldom do they have a history of long-standing psychiatric problems. Rather, most of their symptoms reflect their current condition.

In one commonly encountered scenario, a patient is seen at a chronic pain center after being injured at a job that requires heavy lifting and bending. The person may have experienced a sudden pain while lifting a particularly heavy object. During a few months of rest and recovery, the individual may have believed that the "muscle strain" would heal itself. After months or years of being evaluated by physicians and other health care professionals and after unsuccessful attempts to return to work, the person begins to show signs of considerable emotional distress, including depression, anxiety, and anger. Often these emotional signs are accompanied by feelings of helplessness, low self-esteem, and isolation. Although chronic pain patients may exhibit certain personality traits that potentially contribute to their inability to cope with a chronic disabling condition, rarely are these traits suggestive of significant psychopathology. For these reasons, traditional assessment techniques, particularly projective tests such as the Thematic Apperception Test (TAT) and Rorschach, are not appropriate for the evaluation of chronic pain patients. Rather, measures that more reliably assess the degree of reactive emotional stress are in order.

Certain questions need to be asked about any self-report measure used to assess chronic pain. The first is whether the measure is reliable. Reliability is the degree of consistency and the extent to which a measure is correlated with itself. The second is whether the measure is valid. Validity is the degree to which an instrument measures what it is supposed to measure and the extent to which it is correlated with other known measures. Using a psychometric measure can be likened to shooting at a target. If a test is reliable, it will hit close to the same spot every time. If a test is valid, it will hit the spot that it is supposed to hit. Ideally, a reliable and valid measure will assess a certain area in the same way and with acceptable accuracy every time it is used.

A third question is whether the measure is clinically useful and appropriate. Although a test may be recognized as a "good" measure, it may not assess what is most important. The clinician needs first to identify the most important constructs (e.g., depression, functional capacity) and then find a measure (or measures) that will best evaluate those constructs.

Lastly, it is important to know how easily the measure can be administered, scored, and interpreted. Some questionnaires are completed and sent off to be scored electronically. Interpretations of the results are computer-driven and often reflect the purpose for which the test was originally designed. A test designed to measure psychopathology may have only limited utility in identifying candidates for treatment. Moreover, some patients may become defensive because they do not understand the reasons for completing lengthy personality tests that seem unrelated to their condition. Ideally, personnel trained in issues related to chronic pain will administer, score, and interpret psychometric tests used in assessing chronic pain. A consideration of the components of the pain experience listed in Table 3.1 (p. 19) can be useful in predicting the efficacy of a given treatment. A worthwhile goal is to establish specific criteria in each of these areas that will help identify the best candidates for specific pain therapies.

TYPES OF
PSYCHOMETRIC MEASURES

PAIN INTENSITY SCALES

One of the primary goals of treatment for chronic pain is obviously to decrease the intensity of the pain. As a result, it is important to monitor pain intensity both for a period before treatment and throughout the course of treatment. The numerous ways to measure pain intensity include numerical pain ratings, visual analogue scales, verbal rating scales, pain drawings, and a combination of standardized questionnaires.

The daily monitoring of pain intensity over a 1- to 2-week period before the start of therapy has a number of benefits. First, more information is obtained than can be gained from a single index of perceived pain intensity. More specifically, averaging multiple measures of pain intensity over time increases the reliability and validity of the assessment and is preferable to a single rating of pain intensity. Second, average pain intensity ratings can serve as a baseline to help establish whether continued treatment is needed after an appropriate trial period. Baseline measures are essential to judgments

**TABLE 3.1: ASSESSMENT CATEGORIES AND
FREQUENTLY USED PSYCHOMETRIC MEASURES**

1. **Psychosocial History**
    Comprehensive Pain Questionnaire
    CAGE Questionnaire
    Michigan Alcoholism Screening Test (MAST)
    Self-Administered Alcoholism Screen Test (SAAST)
    Structured Clinical Interview for *DSM-IV*

2. **Pain Intensity**
    Numerical rating scales
    Visual analogue scales
    Verbal rating scales
    Pain drawings

3. **Mood and Personality**
    Minnesota Multiphasic Personality Inventory (MMPI)
    Symptom Checklist 90 (SCL-90)
    Millon Behavior Health Inventory (MBHI)
    Illness Behavior Questionnaire (IBQ)
    Beck Depression Inventory (BDI)

4. **Pain Beliefs and Coping**
    Coping Strategies Questionnaire (CSQ)
    Pain Management Inventory (PMI)
    Pain Self-Efficacy Questionnaire (PSEQ)
    Survey of Pain Attitudes (SOPA)
    Inventory of Negative Thoughts in Response to Pain (INTRP)

5. **Functional Capacity**
    Sickness Impact Profile (SIP)
    Short-Form Health Survey (SF-36)
    Multidimensional Pain Inventory (MPI)
    Pain Disability Index (PDI)

6. **Medication Monitoring**
    Medication record
    Monitoring devices

7. **Adverse Effects**
    Adverse Effects Checklist

about the overall impact of treatment for pain. Pain intensity rating methods have evolved from designs originally developed by Thomas Budzynski (Budzynski et al., 1973) and by Ronald Melzack (Melzack, 1975). A number of studies have shown that self-monitored pain intensity ratings are both reliable and valid.

Numerical pain ratings often involve the patient's rating of his or her pain on a scale of 0 to 10 or 0 to 100. Ideally, the external validity of the measure is improved by descriptive anchors that help the patient understand the meaning of each numerical value. Another popular means of measuring pain intensity is the visual analogue scale, which uses a straight line (often 10 cm. long) with extreme limits of pain at either end. The pain patient is instructed to place a mark at the point on the line that best indicates present pain severity. Scores are obtained by measuring the distance from the end labeled "no pain" to the mark provided by the patient. Evidence exists for the validity of the visual analogue scale. The disadvantages of this method are that it is time-consuming to score and that its validity for older patients is questionable.

There are a number of verbal rating scales (Table 3.2, p. 21). These scales consist of terms (as few as 4 or as many as 15, often ranked in order of severity from "no pain" to "excruciating pain") that are chosen by patients to describe their pain. Verbal scales not only measure pain intensity but also assess sensory and reactive dimensions of the pain experience. Patients choose words from a list of pain descriptors that best describe their pain (e.g., piercing, stabbing, shooting, burning, throbbing).

Of all of the self-report measures, numerical rating scales are most popular. However, there is no evidence that visual analogue scales or verbal rating scales are any less sensitive in measuring changes due to treatment. All of these measures have been shown to be acceptable in the quantification of clinical pain.

The McGill Pain Questionnaire (MPQ; Melzack, 1975) is a popular comprehensive questionnaire that includes 20 subclasses of descriptors as well as a numerical pain intensity scale and a dermatome pain drawing. A short form of the McGill Questionnaire has also been published (Melzack, 1987; see pp. 33-34). The MPQ measures different aspects of the pain experience and is sensitive to treatment effects and differential diagnosis.

MOOD AND PERSONALITY MEASURES

The presence of psychopathology and/or extreme emotionality has been seen as a contraindication for certain therapies. There is ongoing debate among mental health professionals about the best way to measure psychopathology and/or emotional distress in chronic pain patients. Most measures are helpful in ruling out severe psychiatric disturbance. Unfortunately, no measure can boast validity in accurately predicting treatment outcome. The measures most commonly used to evaluate personality and emotional distress include the Minnesota Multiphasic Personality Inventory (MMPI; Hathaway et al.,

---

TABLE 3.2: EXAMPLES OF VERBAL RATING SCALES OF PAIN INTENSITY

1. No pain	1. None	1. No pain	1. Not noticeable
2. Mild	2. Mild	2. Mild	2. Just noticeable
3. Moderate	3. Moderate	3. Discomforting	3. Very weak
4. Severe	4. Severe	4. Distressing	4. Weak
	5. Very Severe	5. Horrible	5. Mild
		6. Excruciating	6. Moderate
			7. Strong
			8. Intense
			9. Very strong
			10. Severe
			11. Very intense
			12. Excruciating

1989), the Symptom Checklist 90 (SCL-90-R; Derogotis, 1977, 1983), the Millon Behavior Health Inventory (MBHI; Millon, Green, & Meagher, 1979), the Illness Behavior Questionnaire (IBQ; Pilowsky & Spence, 1975), and the Beck Depression Inventory (BDI; Beck & Steer, 1987).

The MMPI is the most popular instrument used in assessing chronic pain patients. This measure consists of 561 true-false items and yields distinct profiles of pain patients. Studies have shown that these profiles can predict return to work in males as well as response to surgical treatment in both genders. The revised version now in use (MMPI-2) replicates the profile patterns of the original MMPI. This test is widely used to measure psychopathology; however, when used with chronic pain patients, the profiles can be misinterpreted because of the physical symptoms frequently endorsed by these patients.

The SCL-90 is a 90-item checklist with a 5-point scale that offers a global index score as well as 9 subscale scores. The SCL-90 is used for the general assessment of emotional distress. It is a relatively brief measure and better accepted by pain patients. It is easy to inspect individual items that may pertain specifically to persons with chronic pain. The disadvantages of this measure are that all subscales are highly correlated and that there are no validity scales to indicate the presence of subtle inconsistencies in responses.

The MBHI, another popular measure for assessing mood and personality, includes 150 true-false items and offers 20 subscales that measure (a) styles relating to providers, (b) psychosocial stressors, and (c) response to illness. The advantage of the MBHI is that the scales are not subject to misinterpretation due to physical symptoms. Unlike other measures, the MBHI emphasizes medical rather than emotional concerns.

The IBQ is commonly used to evaluate emotionality and illness behavior in chronic pain patients. This questionnaire includes 62 true-false items and consists of 7 subscales measuring symptoms and abnormal illness-related behavior. Patients who are not known to have organic pathology that would account for their pain tend to have higher IBQ scores. The IBQ is also correlated with anxiety measures.

The BDI assesses depressive symptoms in chronic pain patients. This 21-item self-report questionnaire measures the severity of depression and is commonly used to evaluate the outcome of treatment. It is easy to administer and score. One limitation is the potential for misinterpretation of an elevated depression score as a result of the frequent endorsement of somatic items (e.g., fatigue, sleep disturbances, and loss of sexual interest) by chronic pain patients.

BELIEFS AND COPING SCALES

Pain perception is important in predicting the outcome of treatment. Unrealistic or negative thoughts about an ongoing pain problem may contribute to increased pain and emotional distress, decreased functioning, and greater reliance on medication. Certain chronic pain patients are prone to maladaptive beliefs about their condition that may not be compatible with the physical nature of their pain (e.g., "My pain is getting worse - eventually it will take over my entire body, and I will become completely handicapped"). Patients with adequate psychological functioning exhibit a greater tendency to ignore their pain, use coping self-statements (e.g., "I can get through this"), and remain active in order to divert their attention from their pain.

A number of self-report measures assess coping and pain attitudes. These measures are particularly useful in evaluating pain perception. The most popular tests used to measure coping style and maladaptive beliefs include the Coping Strategies Questionnaire (CSQ; Rosenstiel & Keefe, 1983), the Pain Management Inventory (PMI; Brown, Nicassio, & Wallston, 1989), the Pain Self-Efficacy Questionnaire (PSEQ; Lorig et al., 1989), the Survey of Pain Attitudes (SOPA; Jensen, Karoly, & Huger, 1987), and the Inventory of Negative Thoughts in Response to Pain (INTRP; Gil et al., 1990). Patients who have a high score on the Catastrophizing Scale of the CSQ, who endorse passive coping on the PMI, who demonstrate low self-efficacy regarding their ability to manage their pain on the PSEQ, who describe themselves as disabled by their pain on the SOPA, and who report frequent negative thoughts about their pain on the INTRP are at greatest risk for poor treatment outcome. It is suspected that patients who have unrealistic beliefs and expectations about their condition (e.g., "I will eventually find someone who will properly diagnose and fix my pain problem") are also poor candidates for pain treatment.

FUNCTIONAL CAPACITY MEASURES

Some clinicians consider pain reduction meaningless if there is no noticeable change in function. Thus, some reliable measurement of functional capacity before the initiation of therapy should be used. A noticeable increase in level of activity helps to justify continued therapy. A number of measures can be used to assess activity level and function. These include the Sickness Impact Profile (SIP; Bergner et al., 1981), the Short-Form Health Survey (SF-36; Ware & Sherbourne, 1992), the Multidimensional Pain Inventory (MPI; Kerns, Turk, & Rudy, 1985), and the Pain Disability Index (PDI; Pollard, 1984).

The SIP is a 136-item checklist with 12 subscales measuring levels of physical and psychosocial functioning. Each item is weighted, and the scales are correlated with other functional capacity measures. Shorter versions of the SIP (e.g., the Roland and Morris Disability Questionnaire [Roland & Morris, 1983]) are suitable for the assessment of function in chronic pain patients.

The SF-36, which was initially developed from the Medical Outcomes Study to survey health status, includes 8 scales that measure (a) limitations in physical activities due to health problems, (b) limitations in social activities due to physical and emotional problems, (c) limitations in usual role activities due to physical health problems, (d) bodily pain, (e) general mental health, (f) limitations in usual role activities due to emotional problems, (g) vitality (energy and fatigue), and (h) general health perceptions. The SF-36 is favored over the SIP because it is a shorter test with excellent reliability and validity. The SIP is preferred if the population being evaluated includes patients with extreme physical limitations.

The MPI is a 56-item measure made up of 7-point rating scales. The subscales assess activity interference, perceived support, pain severity, negative mood, and perceived control. The advantage of this self-report instrument is that it was created specifically for chronic pain patients and can be useful in classifying those patients into three types: dysfunctional, interpersonally distressed, and adaptive copers.

Other functional measures include the Oswestry Disability Questionnaire (Fairbank et al., 1980), the Chronic Illness Problem Inventory (Kames et al., 1984), the Waddell Disability Instrument (Waddell & Main, 1984), and the Functional Rating Scale (Evans & Kagan, 1986). Automated measurement devices, such as the portable up-time calculator and the pedometer, are useful in obtaining accurate measures of activity. These devices should be used in conjunction with self-monitoring assessment techniques.

BEHAVIORAL ANALYSIS

A thorough behavioral analysis is important in the successful rehabilitation of each chronic pain patient. Wilbert Fordyce (Fordyce, 1976), one of the early proponents of behavioral assessment, put forward the learning theory of chronic pain. Basically, he highlighted the important distinction between what pain patients say and what they do. Thus, instead of relying solely on subjective measures of chronic pain, investigators should also evaluate objective, observable manifestations of how the patient responds to pain. A significant component of the learning theory of chronic pain is to distinguish between "well" behaviors and "pain" behaviors. Further, it is essential to identify factors that perpetuate pain behaviors.

The first step in behavioral analysis is to identify overt pain-related behaviors in pain patients. These may include posturing, limping, requests for pain medication, and reliance on cervical collars, back braces, canes, and so forth. All of these behaviors are observable and tend to perpetuate a disability identity. Other measures used in a behavioral analysis include self-monitored observations and automated devices. One measurement method that has been shown to be both reliable and valid has been put forward by Dr. Francis Keefe (Keefe & Block, 1982). Pain patients are videotaped while they are asked to sit, recline, stand, and walk. The videotapes are rated by independent observers with regard to guarding, bracing, rubbing, grimacing, and sighing. For a new patient at a chronic pain center, the videotape session serves as a baseline against which to evaluate progress. Additional methods have been incorporated into the behavioral analysis of chronic pain patients, including a problem-oriented approach to the assessment of pain medication use and an observational approach to the assessment of daily activity.

SUMMARY

In summary, there are many dimensions to chronic pain, and the categories of pain intensity, emotional distress, functional capacity, pain beliefs, medication usage, and psychosocial history need to be assessed both prior to and during participation in a pain management program.

SEMISTRUCTURED INTERVIEW

Although self-report psychometric tests may be reliable and valid for assessment of the pain experience, the most popular means of evaluating the psychological state of the patient is a semistructured interview. Pertinent information acquired during an interview is frequently given significant weight when a decision regarding treatment is made. Before meeting with the patient, it is helpful to review all referral information, including discharge summaries, psychological testing results, the notes of the patient's previous physician(s), and medical history reports. It is also important to recognize that some pain patients may not be eager to admit to the emotional component of their pain. For this and other reasons, it is crucial to establish a comfortable rapport with each patient at the beginning of the first visit.

The following areas should be covered during the initial interview: (a) pain history; (b) pain description; (c) aggravating factors; (d) past and current treatments; (e) activity level/work status; (f) social history/emotional support system; (g) psychological factors; and (h) motivation to change behavior.

The goal is to identify "red flags" in each of these areas. Rating each category as positive or negative to signify the presence or absence of a problem can alert the clinician to difficulties that the patient may be encountering.

1. *Relevant Medical History.* The first part of the interview elicits information regarding the history of the patient's pain. Asking what previous physicians have said about the pain is often a helpful way to begin. It is also informative to ask what the patient believes is the chief cause of the pain. Additional information about onset of the pain and the patient's medical history can be valuable. The clinician should be alerted to those cases in which the patient is seriously worried that previous physicians might have missed something important or in which the patient is having particular difficulty in understanding and accepting the condition involved.

2. *Pain Description.* The second part of the interview is concerned with the description of the pain, its intensity, and its pattern. The patient is asked whether the pain is worse in the morning, afternoon, or evening or if its intensity can be predicted with any degree of consistency. Information on sleep patterns is also obtained. Special attention should be given to those patients who are unable to predict fluctuations in their pain and who feel that they have little control over their lives because of this unpredictability.

3. *Aggravating Factors.* Patients are asked to identify factors that make their pain worse or better. Patients who identify multiple aggravating factors and who report that their pain interferes significantly with their lives, leaving them with little sense of control, are identified as possibly needing a behavioral management approach.

4. *Past and Current Treatments.* The usefulness of medications and other treatments in controlling the patient's pain should be discussed. Information not only about what treatments have been tried but also about how much the patient understands those treatments is important. Patients who are convinced that only medical interventions can help them may not be good candidates for a behaviorally based program.

5. *Activity Level/Work Status.* The patient's activity level and current work status should be discussed. The patient is asked to describe a typical day of activity. The clinician should be alerted when a patient is unemployed, reports reclining

and being in bed much of the day, and/or cites extreme reluctance to be active. Information about pacing and management on both good and bad days should be noted.

6. *Social History/Emotional Support System.*   If not already recorded, relevant biographical data should be obtained, including marital status, educational level, occupational and vocational status, and any pertinent information about members of the patient's immediate family. Much of this information can be obtained when the patient completes the Comprehensive Pain Questionnaire (see pp. 35-43). Information also should be obtained on the patient's perception of the level of outside support available to him or her in dealing with chronic pain. Patients who suggest ongoing conflict and disharmony at home and who report minimal support from family members or significant others need to be identified. The interviewer must ascertain whether the family reinforces pain behaviors and whether these behaviors act as discriminative cues for further display of pain. In this regard, it is important to interview at least one close family member.

7. *Psychological Factors.* Relevant psychological factors, the patient's mental status, and in particular the patient's level of emotional distress must be assessed. Patients are asked to report their level of depression, anxiety, irritability, and overall well-being in dealing with their pain. In addition, they are asked whether they feel life is worth living or whether they have had any suicidal ideations. Any history of psychiatric or psychological evaluations and/or treatment or history of suicide attempts should be noted. Results from the MMPI, SCL-90, BDI, and other psychometric measures can be helpful. The clinicians should be alerted when a patient reports a great deal of emotional distress related to the pain. History of drug, alcohol, and sexual abuse should also be obtained. Structured-interview measures have been published for the assessment of alcoholism and drug abuse (e.g., the CAGE Questionnaire [Ewings, 1984; Mayfield, McLeod, & Hall, 1974], the Michigan Alcoholism Screening Test [MAST; Selzer, 1971], and the Self-Administered Alcoholism Screen Test [SAAST; Swenson & Morse, 1975]) and for psychiatric diagnosis (the Structured Clinical Interview for *DSM* [SCID; Williams et al., 1992]).

8. *Motivation to Change Behavior.* In evaluating a patient's general motivation, it is useful to ask what they would be doing differently if they did not have any pain. Factors to be noted include previous job satisfaction, compensation status, future vocational options, and present willingness to participate actively in a rehabilitation program to help manage pain. Although most patients will state that they would do anything to be the way they were before their pain developed, many are unwilling to take responsibility for the treatment of their

pain. The interviewer should identify those patients who have litigation pending and who seem unwilling to learn to live with their pain. Current research is under way in identifying stages of change of chronic pain which would help in determining readiness for treatment.

Once a patient meets the inclusion criteria for a pain management program, a preapproval letter should be sent to the referring physician or insurance carrier (see Sample Preapproval Request Letter on p. 45). For those persons involved in ongoing litigation, a lien agreement may also be sent and signed (see Sample Lien Agreement on p. 47).

TREATMENT PLAN
AND PATIENT CONTRACT

Patients should be encouraged to create a treatment plan with specific goals. The topics encompassed by the plan may include education, pain monitoring, relaxation training, biofeedback, individual psychotherapy, group therapy, vocational counseling, exercise physiology, and participation in a structured, multidisciplinary program with special emphasis on the most problematic areas. A sample "patient contract" drawn up prior to enrollment in a structured program is included on page 13.

Throughout the course of the pain management program, contract goals should be reviewed and updated. It is useful to distribute a list of the combined goals to all members of the group. Goals which are either unobtainable or unrealistic can be challenged by the other group members. Halfway through the program the members should be asked for a report of how well they are meeting their goals. The goals should be included in any discharge summary and be consulted for each person on follow-up. An example of an initial psychological report is presented on pages 49-51.

PATIENT EXCLUSION CRITERIA

There are a number of reasons to exclude a patient from participating in a structured pain program. These include the following:

1. The patient shows significant anger, disruptive pain behavior, or negative affect. Patients who are in crisis and need ongoing supportive therapy may not benefit from a group experience.
2. The patient is markedly different from the other group members in terms of pain site, pain intensity, or disposition. Structured, time-limited programs seem to be most successful when the group is homogeneous.

3. The patient is unwilling to accept a rehabilitation model for the management of pain. He or she may expect that a suitable medical treatment will eventually be offered to resolve the pain. As a result, he or she may lack the motivation to participate fully in a pain management program.

4. The patient demonstrates limited intelligence. Individuals with markedly poor reading skills and an inability to grasp basic concepts of rehabilitation will be at a distinct disadvantage.

5. The patient has a severe physical handicap that makes ambulation and/or sitting for up to an hour extremely difficult.

6. The patient has a history of alcohol or medication abuse. Patients should be carefully screened and may be excluded if an ongoing addiction is found.

7. The patient violates a mutually agreed upon contract.

8. The patient is coerced to attend the pain program. Patients who attend of their own free will are the most successful.

MEDICAL EVALUATION FORM*

Name: _____ Age: _____ Date: _____

Medical Record # _____

Referring Physician: _____

Chief Complaint: _____

Problem List: _____

HISTORY OF PRESENT ILLNESS (separate history for each pain problem)

1. Time since onset of pain and circumstances of onset:

2. Temporal characteristics:

3. Statement of intensity:

4. Statement of character:

5. What exacerbates or relieves:

6. Associated symptoms (numbness, weakness, incontinence, other):

7. Prior treatments and effects:

PSYCHOSOCIAL HISTORY

1. Work history:

---

*This Medical Evaluation Form was initially created by Nathaniel Katz, MD (unpublished).

2. Activities:

3. Ongoing litigation/compensation:

4. Sleep habits:

5. Family life:

6. Psychological symptoms (depression, anxiety, anger):

MEDICAL HISTORY:

SOCIAL HISTORY:

FAMILY HISTORY (migraines, back pain, suicide, psychiatric, illness, etc.)**:**

ALLERGIES:

MEDICATIONS:

ALCOHOL/ILLICIT DRUGS (CAGE: Have you ever had to *C*ut down your use of a substance? Have others *A*nnoyed you by asking you to do so? Have you felt *G*uilty about using a substance? Have you ever needed an *E*ye-opener?):

TOBACCO:

PHYSICAL EXAMINATION

1. General appearance:

2. General examination (appropriate to the body part or system involved: What maneuvers reproduce the patient's pain? Evidence of trigger points? Nerve damage?):

3. Musculoskeletal examination (range of motion, muscle tenderness or spasm, joint exam, spinal exam):

4. Neurologic examination (as pertinent: mental status, cranial nerve, strength, reflexes, sensation, gait):

LABORATORY FINDINGS:

RADIOGRAPHIC STUDIES:

ASSESSMENT (for each pain problem)

1. Mechanism (somatic, visceral, neuropathic):

2. Etiology (tumor, infection, etc.):

3. Psychological features (depression, litigation, etc.):

4. Physical rehabilitation issues (deconditioned, bed bound, etc.):

PLAN OF CARE:

MCGILL PAIN QUESTIONNAIRE - SHORT FORM*

Directions: Please read each word below, and decide whether it describes what your pain has felt like over the PAST 4 WEEKS. If a word does not describe your pain, circle *NO* (DOES NOT APPLY), and go on to the next item. If a word does describe your pain, then rate how strongly you have felt that sensation (1 = Mild, 2 = Moderate, 3 = Severe). Remember, make these ratings as to how your pain has felt over the PAST 4 WEEKS.

My pain felt like it was . . .	*DOES NOT APPLY*	*MILD*	*MODERATE*	*SEVERE*
1. THROBBING	NO	1	2	3
2. SHOOTING	NO	1	2	3
3. STABBING	NO	1	2	3
4. SHARP	NO	1	2	3
5. CRAMPING	NO	1	2	3
6. GNAWING	NO	1	2	3
7. HOT - BURNING	NO	1	2	3
8. ACHING	NO	1	2	3
9. HEAVY	NO	1	2	3
10. TENDER	NO	1	2	3
11. SPLITTING	NO	1	2	3
12. TIRING - EXHAUSTING	NO	1	2	3
13. SICKENING	NO	1	2	3
14. FEARFUL	NO	1	2	3
15. PUNISHING - CRUEL	NO	1	2	3

Please circle the number which describes your level of pain right now:

0	1	2	3	4	5	6	7	8	9	10
No Pain					Moderate Pain					Worst Pain Possible

Please circle the number which describes your typical level of pain:

0	1	2	3	4	5	6	7	8	9	10
No Pain					Moderate Pain					Worst Pain Possible

*Note. From the "Short-Form McGill Pain Questionnaire," by R. Melzack, 1987, *Pain, 30,* pp. 191-197. Copyright © 1987 by Elsevier Science Publishers. Reprinted with permission.

Please check the word that best describes your pain right now:

- ❐ NO PAIN   ❐ DISTRESSING
- ❐ MILD   ❐ HORRIBLE
- ❐ DISCOMFORTING   ❐ EXCRUCIATING

COMPREHENSIVE
PAIN QUESTIONNAIRE

Please complete this form before your first appointment with the Pain Management Center. Your careful answers will help us to understand your pain problem and design the best treatment program for you.

You may feel concerned about what happens to the information you provide, as much of it is personal. Our records are strictly confidential. No outsider is permitted to see your case record without your written permission.

BACKGROUND INFORMATION

1. Today's date: _____

2. Patient's full name: _____

3. Address: _____

4. Home phone: Area code _____   Number_____

5. Work phone: Area code _____   Number_____

6. Person to contact in an emergency: _____

   Address/Phone number: _____

   _____

7. Sex: ❏ Male   ❏ Female

8. Age: _____   Date of birth: _____

9. Height: _____   Weight: _____

10. Referring physician's name: _____

11. Approximately how far is your home from our office? _____

12. Education (please check all that apply and write number of years completed):

   Years of formal education: _____

   ❏ High school graduate
   ❏ College graduate
   ❏ Advanced degree . . . What degree? _____

13.   Marital status (please check current status):

    ❐ Single (never married)
    ❐ Married . . . How long? _____
    ❐ Remarried . . . How long? _____
    ❐ Separated . . . How long? _____
    ❐ Divorced . . . How long? _____
    ❐ Widowed . . . How long? _____

    If married, please give your spouse's occupation: _____

14.   Number of children: _____   Number of grandchildren: _____

15.   With whom are you currently living (please check all that apply)?

    ❐ Alone
    ❐ Parent
    ❐ Spouse
    ❐ Other(s) . . . Who? _____
    ❐ Children . . . How many live with you? _____

16.   Current occupation or last job: _____

17.   Current employment status (please check all that apply):

    ❐ Employed full-time
    ❐ Employed part-time
    ❐ Unemployed
    ❐ Homemaker
    ❐ Retired
    ❐ Student
    ❐ Unemployed because of pain

18.   Are you currently working?

    ❐ Yes . . . please skip to question 24.   ❐ No . . . Go to question 19.

19.   Would you return to work if you had no pain problem? ❐ Yes   ❐ No

20.   Have you tried to return to work? ❐ Yes   ❐ No

21.   Is your present or previous job still open to you? ❐ Yes   ❐ No

22.   What was your last day of work? Month _____   Day _____   Year _____

23.   Has your employer been helpful and understanding about your pain problem?

    ❐ Yes   ❐ No   ❐ Not applicable

24. Are you receiving compensation or disability payments now? ☐ Yes ☐ No

    If yes, are payments adequate? ☐ Yes ☐ No

25. Do you have an application for compensation or disability payments pending?

    ☐ Yes ☐ No

26. Is your pain the result of an accident? ☐ Yes ☐ No

    If yes, where did it occur? Circle one: home, work, vacation, car, other (describe):

    _____

27. Are you suing anyone because of your pain or injury? ☐ Yes ☐ No

28. Have you brought suit in the past? ☐ Yes ☐ No

    If yes, what was the outcome? _____

CHARACTERISTICS OF PAIN

29. What is the main problem for which you are seeking treatment at the Pain Management Center?

    _____

    _____

30. Please describe the location(s) of your pain:

    _____

31. How long have you had your current pain problem (in years and/or months)?

    _____

32. How did your current pain start? Was there a precipitating event?

    _____

    _____

33. How often do you have your pain (please check one)?

    ☐ Constantly (100% of the time)
    ☐ Nearly constantly (60% to 95% of the time)
    ☐ Intermittently (30% to 60% of the time)
    ☐ Occasionally (less than 30% of the time)

34. Please mark the location(s) of your pain on the diagrams below with an "X." If whole areas are
     painful, please shade in the painful area.

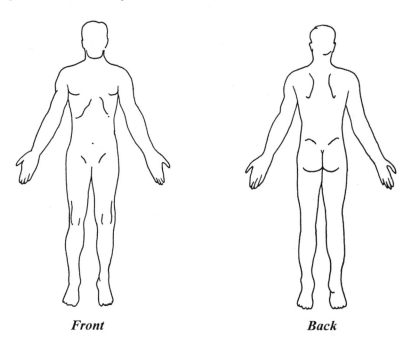

Front   *Back*

35. In general, during the past month when has your pain been the worst (please check one)?

     ❐ Morning   ❐ Afternoon   ❐ Evening   ❐ Night   ❐ No typical pattern

36. How do the following affect your pain (please check one for each item)?

	Decrease	**No Effect**	**Increase**
Lying down	❐	❐	❐
Standing	❐	❐	❐
Sitting	❐	❐	❐
Walking	❐	❐	❐
Exercise (if applicable)	❐	❐	❐
Medication	❐	❐	❐
Relaxation	❐	❐	❐
Thinking about something else	❐	❐	❐
Coughing/Sneezing	❐	❐	❐
Urination	❐	❐	❐
Bowel movements	❐	❐	❐

Are there other factors that make your pain . . .

❐ better (please list)? _____

❐ worse (please list)? _____

37. During the past month, how much did pain interfere with the following activities (circle the number for each item that best describes your situation)?

	Not at all	A little bit	Moder- ately	Quite a bit	Ex- tremely
Going to work	1	2	3	4	5
Performing household chores	1	2	3	4	5
Doing yard work or shopping	1	2	3	4	5
Socializing with friends	1	2	3	4	5
Participating in recreation	1	2	3	4	5
Having sexual relations	1	2	3	4	5
Physically exercising	1	2	3	4	5
Sleeping	1	2	3	4	5
Eating	1	2	3	4	5

38. How often during the day do you lie down because of pain?

❏ Never   ❏ Seldom   ❏ Sometimes   ❏ Often   ❏ Constantly

39. Which of the following best describes your usual level of pain?

❏ Mild   ❏ Uncomfortable   ❏ Distressing   ❏ Very Severe   ❏ Unbearable

40. Please rate your pain intensity on a scale from 0 = no pain to 10 = excruciating, incapacitating, worst pain possible.

Write the *number* in the spaces below:

Describes your pain at its worst   _____
Describes your pain at its least   _____
Describes your pain on the average   _____

41. When you are in pain, how often is your husband/wife/other family member supportive and encouraging?

❏ Never   ❏ Seldom   ❏ Sometimes   ❏ Frequently   ❏ Always

42. When you are in pain, how often does your husband/wife/other family member ignore you or become angry?

❏ Never   ❏ Seldom   ❏ Sometimes   ❏ Frequently   ❏ Always

43. How often has there been disharmony/conflict between you and your spouse, parent or children since the start of your pain?

❏ Never   ❏ Seldom   ❏ Sometimes   ❏ Frequently   ❏ Always

44. During the past month, how often have you been tense or anxious?

    ❏ Never   ❏ Seldom   ❏ Sometimes   ❏ Frequently   ❏ Always

45. During the past month, how often have you been depressed or discouraged?

    ❏ Never   ❏ Seldom   ❏ Sometimes   ❏ Frequently   ❏ Always

46. During the past month, how often have you been irritable and upset?

    ❏ Never   ❏ Seldom   ❏ Sometimes   ❏ Frequently   ❏ Always

47. Have any of your family members ever had a chronic pain problem? ❏ Yes   ❏ No

    If yes, who? _____

    What kind of pain? _____

PAIN TREATMENT

48. Please check all of the treatments you have tried for your pain, and complete the appropriate columns at the right.

Treatment	*Dates*	*Results*
❏ Hospital bed rest	_____	_____
❏ Traction	_____	_____
❏ Surgery	_____	_____
❏ Hypnosis	_____	_____
❏ Acupuncture	_____	_____
❏ Nerve block or injection	_____	_____
❏ TENS (electrical stimulator)	_____	_____
❏ Physical therapy	_____	_____
❏ Exercise	_____	_____
❏ Heat treatment	_____	_____
❏ Biofeedback	_____	_____
❏ Psychotherapy	_____	_____
❏ Chiropractic	_____	_____
❏ Other	_____	_____

49. Have you ever had psychiatric, psychological, or social work evaluations or treatments for any problem, including your current pain? ❏ Yes   ❏ No

    If yes, when? _____

50.   In the past year, has your weight (check one)

    ❐ Remained the same?
    ❐ Increased? By how many pounds?_____
    ❐ Decreased? By how many pounds? _____

    If your weight decreased were you dieting? ❐ Yes   ❐ No

51.   Do you smoke cigarettes? ❐ Yes   ❐ No

    If yes, how many packs a day? _____   For how many years? _____

52.   Do you drink alcoholic beverages? ❐ Yes   ❐ No

    If yes, what/how much? _____ How often? _____

53.   Please check all of the medications you have tried for your current pain problem, and complete
    the appropriate columns at right.

Medication	Drug Name	Approximate Dates (Start/Stop)	Daily Dose
❐ Aspirin	_____	_____	_____
❐ Acetaminophen	_____	_____	_____
❐ Nonsteroidal anti-inflammatories (e.g., Motrin, Naprosyn, Indocin, Feldene)	_____	_____	_____
❐ Antidepressants (e.g., Elavil, Desyrel, Nardil, Tofranil, Sinequan)	_____	_____	_____
❐ Codeine (or products containing codeine)	_____	_____	_____
❐ Oral narcotics (e.g., Percocet, Darvocet, Dilaudid Talwin)	_____	_____	_____
❐ Injectable narcotics (e.g., Morphine, Demerol)	_____	_____	_____
❐ Barbiturates (e.g., Nembutal, Seconal)	_____	_____	_____
❐ Tranquilizers (e.g., Valium, Librium, Xanax)	_____	_____	_____

Medication	*Drug Name*	*Approximate Dates (Start/Stop)*	*Daily Dose*
❏ Muscle relaxants (e.g. Robaxin, Flexeril, Baclofen)	_____	_____	_____
❏ Major tranquil-izers (e.g., Thora-zine, Haldol)	_____	_____	_____
❏ Sleeping medi-cation (e.g., Dalmane, Restoril, chloral hydrate)	_____	_____	_____

54. Aside from your pain problem, how is your general health (please check one)?

❏ Excellent   ❏ Minor health problems only   ❏ Major health problems

55. Have you had any of the following health problems (please check all that apply)?

❏ High blood pressure   ❏ Diabetes or high blood sugar
❏ Angina or chest pain   ❏ Kidney disease
❏ Heart attack   ❏ Liver disease
❏ Asthma or wheezing   ❏ Tumor-induced angiogenesis (TIA) or stroke
❏ Chronic cough   ❏ Seizure or epilepsy
❏ Bleeding problem   ❏ Cancer
❏ Arthritis   ❏ Other; specify _____

56. Are there things causing stress in your life other than your current pain problem?

❏ Yes   ❏ No

If yes, please describe: _____
_____
_____

57. What medications are you taking (other than those you have listed for your pain problem)?

_____

58. Do you have any allergies?

_____

59.   Surgeries:

Date	Hospital	Type of Operation	Type of Anesthesia
_____	_____	_____	_____
_____	_____	_____	_____
_____	_____	_____	_____
_____	_____	_____	_____
_____	_____	_____	_____

60.   What are you expecting from treatment at the pain center? Is there any additional information you think we should have?

_____

_____

_____

_____

_____

_____

_____

_____

_____

SAMPLE PREAPPROVAL
REQUEST LETTER

April 22, 1996

Knicely Dunn, RN, CCM
Utilization Review Nurse
Generic Insurance Company
100 Main Street
Dover, NH 03820

RE: Ray D. Ator
DOB: 3/29/49
File #: WC 909-876543 F

Dear Ms. Dunn:

I am writing regarding Mr. Ator who is a 47-year-old white male referred to the Pain Management Center by Dr. Justin Hale. He is being evaluated for treatment of persistent headaches and low back pain.

As you may know, Mr. Ator was involved in a work-related accident when he fell off a ladder in 1990. Since then he has been seen by multiple health care professionals and has not responded to traditional medical interventions. I had the opportunity to evaluate him on 12/4/95. Mr. Ator has given me permission to send you a copy of my initial psychological report.

Mr. Ator is being recommended for the 10-week group-based structured pain management program offered at Brigham and Women's Hospital. This is a 1 day per week program designed for persons with chronic pain. The program consists of didactic sessions, relaxation training, and exercise physiology designed to reduce pain, increase coping, and improve physical functioning. We also will address vocational rehabilitation issues. I believe that Mr. Ator would benefit from participation in this program. He has agreed to attend with his wife. They have addressed a number of specific goals for treatment, including reduction in use of medication, increased physical functioning, and reduction in anxiety, depression, and irritability. Mr. Ator has agreed to actively participate in the program. He has also agreed to monitor his pain, activity, mood, and use of medication.

The next 10-week program is scheduled to begin Thursday, June 6, 1996. I am enclosing a program brochure and cost information. Please feel free to contact me if you need additional information to aid in the preapproval process.

Sincerely,

Robert N. Jamison, PhD
Program Director

RNJ/mdd

SAMPLE LIEN AGREEMENT

In consideration of certain health care services that have been or will be provided to me by the Pain Management Center at Brigham and Women's Hospital, I, Rosie Scenario, hereby irrevocably assign all of my rights, title, and interest in and to a portion of all insurance or other proceeds of any type payable to me for charges incurred in connection with my illness or injury to The Anesthesia Foundation. I hereby authorize payment of said proceeds plus costs and interest to BWH Anesthesia Foundation, before any disbursement to me.

_Rosie Scenario_____   _4/16/96_____
Patient Signature   Date

_John Doe_____   _4/16/96_____
Witness Signature   Date

ACCEPTANCE

I, the undersigned attorney for Rosie Scenario, acknowledge the above lien and assignment and agree to pay over to The Anesthesia Foundation any incurred sums, costs, and interest directly from the proceeds of any recovery collected in the above claim for personal injuries.

Attorney Signature		Attorney Name Printed	Date
Street Address			
City	State	Zip	Attorney Telephone
Date of Loss	Defendant		
Insurance Company			Claim Number
Court			Docket Number

SAMPLE INITIAL
PSYCHOLOGICAL REPORT

PRIMARY PAIN COMPLAINTS

1. Bilateral cervical pain
2. Bilateral upper extremity pain
3. History of headaches
4. Bilateral knee pain

BACKGROUND INFORMATION

Mr. Doe is a 39-year-old white male who was referred to the Pain Management Center by Dr. Smith for evaluation and consideration of treatment for his persistent cervical and upper extremity pain. He was referred for participation in the structured pain management program for persons with chronic pain.

Reportedly, Mr. Doe has had arm and neck pain since September 1991. He was employed as an assembly line worker, and his job required heavy lifting of 50-pound containers. Mr. Doe stated that on one occasion he was doing an excessive amount of lifting when he experienced numbness and tingling in both hands and arms. Since that time he has had surgery on both of his elbows and has undergone a neck fusion at C5-C6. Over the past 2 years, he has seen multiple health care professionals and reports that his condition has gradually worsened. He reportedly underwent mylography and had a severe reaction requiring hospitalization. Multiple EMGs of his elbows suggest evidence of pathology. At one point Mr. Doe was diagnosed with thoracic outlet syndrome. He was recently told that he has degenerative disc disease with stenosis and bone spurs in his neck. Mr. Doe has a history of hypertension and has had one period of chest pain. Otherwise, he describes his health as excellent.

PAIN DESCRIPTION

Mr. Doe states that his pain is constant. The pain radiates from his neck into both shoulders, arms, and hands. He also has significant headaches. He rates his pain between 8 and 10 on a scale of 0 to 10 and at times describes it as unbearable.

Mr. Doe has identified factors that aggravate his condition. He reports having difficulty getting comfortable while lying down; he often sleeps in a recliner. He experiences increased pain while standing, sitting, walking, bending, lifting, coughing, and sneezing. He states there is no particular pattern to his pain. He has experienced significant sleep disturbances. In addition, since its onset, his pain has significantly interfered with his ability to perform all activities, including household chores, yard work, shopping, socializing, sexual relations, physical exercise, and appetite. Mr. Doe also notes that rainy weather makes his pain worse.

MEDICATIONS

Mr. Doe has tried a number of different medications for the management of his pain, including Advil, Prozac, Vicodin, and Flexeril. He is currently taking 10 mg. of Prozac once per day, six Vicodin per day, and one Flexeril at night. He hopes that over time he will not need to rely on medication for the management of his pain.

ACTIVITY LEVEL

Mr. Doe is relatively inactive. He states at times he has trouble relaxing. He rarely leaves his home and he is not involved in a regular exercise program. He experiences both an aching pain and a sharp shooting pain, and he says that he can tell the difference between muscle and nerve pain. He has problems pacing himself and is often "in a hurry to get things done." Mr. Doe takes frequent naps during the day and has problems sleeping at night. He is reluctant to perform household chores because these tend to increase his pain.

SOCIAL HISTORY

Mr. Doe has some posthigh school training. He is married and has two children: a son (age 8) and a daughter (age 10). This is the first marriage for both he and his wife. His parents are retired and living in Florida. His father has a history of heart complaints. His mother is diagnosed with noninsulin dependent diabetes. Mr. Doe has two younger sisters and one younger brother. All of his siblings are in good health. No other family member has a pain-related problem. Mr. Doe has an uncle who is an alcoholic. Otherwise there is no history of alcohol or drug abuse problems in his family. Mr. Doe denies any history of sexual abuse in his family.

Mr. Doe has been awarded social security disability and is currently receiving compensation benefits. He is not involved in litigation related to his pain. Mr. Doe states that his family is always supportive and encouraging; however, he admits that at times family members become irritated and that there is disharmony and conflict. Much of this he attributes to guilt feelings and irritability associated with his pain. He describes himself as frequently tense, anxious, and irritable. He also states that he is always depressed and discouraged. Mr. Doe has been evaluated by a psychiatrist in association with his pain. He does not smoke cigarettes or drink alcoholic beverages.

BEHAVIORAL OBSERVATIONS

Mr. Doe was interviewed at the Pain Management Center. He showed no difficulty in walking to the interview room. He appeared to be relaxed. He was verbal, pleasant, oriented, and willing to share information regarding his condition about which he displayed adequate insight. He did not exhibit excessive emotional distress. He stated that he had suicidal ideations in the past because of the intensity of his pain; however, he did not report having any immediate plans to harm himself, and he recognized that some of these feelings were related to his perception of hopelessness about his condition.

Mr. Doe was asked to complete an SCL-90, which is a symptom checklist by which emotional distress is evaluated. A significant elevation on the Global Symptom Index was evident. Elevations were also apparent on the Hostility, Anxiety, Depression, Interpersonal Sensitivity, Obsessionality, and Somatization subscales. Mr. Doe described problems with memory and concentration and said that he felt that others were unsympathetic about his condition. He endorsed items suggesting hopelessness about the future and feelings of worthlessness. He also endorsed items reflecting anxiety stating that he often experiences nervousness and tension associated with his pain. He described temper outbursts that he could not control and urges to break and smash things. During the interview he said he knew that his feelings and behaviors were associated with frustration about his limitations. Overall, Mr. Doe shows considerable emotional distress that may tend to exacerbate his pain.

PAIN CLASSIFICATION

Based on the categories of pain intensity, emotional distress, perceived support, and activity interference, Mr. Doe is classified as a Class III chronic pain patient - Interpersonally Distressed.

DSM-IV Diagnosis: Pain associated with both psychological factors and a general medical condition - chronic (307.89).

RECOMMENDATIONS

Mr. Doe is scheduled for an evaluation by one of the physicians at the Pain Management Center. He is very interested in participating in the structured day treatment program. He says that he benefits from talking about his condition. He has tried a number of different strategies in the past, including relaxation training and individual psychotherapy. However, he is resistant to traditional psychotherapy, feeling that somehow this technique is unrelated to his current condition, and he has had difficulty in concentrating on relaxation strategies.

Mr. Doe would benefit from an educational approach, with a goal of learning to pace his activities and to use cognitive/behavioral techniques to gain a sense of control. Mr. Doe exhibits considerable emotional distress and would also benefit from supportive psychotherapy. He is anxious about his current financial state and his reliance on worker's compensation. Besides the structured group program, vocational rehabilitation and exercise physiology would be beneficial.

The following specific recommendations should be considered:

1. Mr. Doe would benefit from further evaluation of his condition to determine the extent to which medical interventions will be of help and behavioral factors have perpetuated his pain problem. He would benefit from pain monitoring as well as monitoring of activity and mood.
2. Mr. Doe has been reliant on medication for which he has gained a tolerance. A gradual taper of his medications would be recommended.
3. Mr. Doe shows evidence of anxiety and irritability which may exacerbate his pain complaint. He may benefit from relaxation training with EMG and thermal biofeedback.
4. Mr. Doe has recurrent negative thoughts associated with his pain. He would benefit from individual and group cognitive/behavioral therapy designed to help manage his condition despite ongoing discomfort. He would further benefit from patient education and participation in a structured program where he could interact with others to gain a sense of control over his pain.
5. Mr. Doe is very limited physically and has fallen into a pattern of frequent naps and inactivity. A program designed to gradually increase his function and to help him gain confidence in being active throughout the day would be recommended.
6. Mr. Doe has limited transferable skills and seems unable to return to his former place of employment at this time due to his pain. A functional capacity evaluation and assessment with a vocational rehabilitation counselor would be recommended to determine his current level of functioning and to explore options for a return to work.

We will discuss his case as part of the multidisciplinary case conference and will develop a specific treatment plan.

Robert N. Jamison, PhD
Clinical Psychologist

cc: Dr. Smith

CHAPTER 4

Therapy Issues

People respond to people who respond.
Anonymous

GROUP THERAPY

Pain patients frequently show signs of emotional distress, with evidence of depression, anxiety, and irritability. Group therapy with a cognitive/behavioral orientation is designed to help patients gain control of the emotional reactions associated with chronic pain. Specific problem-solving strategies offered during group therapy sessions include (a) identifying maladaptive and negative thoughts, (b) disputing irrational thinking, (c) constructing and repeating positive self-statements, (d) learning distraction techniques, (e) working to prevent future catastrophizing, and (f) examining ways to increase social support. In addition, group therapy presents an opportunity to discuss concerns or problems that patients have in common. Unlike psychotherapists in traditional group sessions, group therapists in a pain management program are encouraged to be active facilitators. They may need to redirect the discussion so that every member has an opportunity to speak and no one individual monopolizes the session. Participants should also be offered individual therapy sessions in which to deal with individual issues.

Certain group members may initially be reluctant to discuss personal problems related to their pain. The group therapist must promote a comfortable atmosphere, preventing other participants from being judgmental or negative. The idea must be conveyed

that people are there to learn from one another and to support one another in gaining
control over pain. Individuals who display negative pain behaviors (e.g., moaning, sighing, grimacing, resting their head on the table, lying on the floor, or arriving late or
leaving early without adequate explanation) should be asked to meet with their case
manager to determine whether this behavior can be changed. To maintain a positive
group atmosphere, it may be necessary to ask participants who exhibit excessive negative
behaviors to leave.

GROUP SIZE AND MEETING ROOM

An optimal number of people for group therapy is six to eight. Larger groups
make control of conversation difficult, while participants in smaller groups do not have
adequate opportunities for interaction with others. Attention should be paid to the ar-
rangement of the room. Some chairs are particularly uncomfortable for persons with
chronic pain. Ideally, the chairs should have arms with suitable cushioning and back
support. Chairs that are either very hard or very soft are not appropriate. Chairs that are
too low to the ground make it difficult to get up and down. Minimal requirements for
a meeting room include privacy, comfortable chairs, ample space, wheelchair (and possibly stretcher) accessibility, a drawing board, and easy access to restrooms and water.
Optional equipment includes a VCR and monitor, an overhead projector, a slide projector,
and a screen.

LEADERSHIP STYLE

Many different leadership styles are useful in facilitating a therapy group. Whatever style is used, the therapist should be flexible enough to tailor that style to the needs
of the particular group involved. Most important, the therapist needs to appear at ease
and comfortable, without seeming artificial or insincere. Research on outcome suggests
that the perceived helpfulness of any structured program is highly related to the relationship between the therapist and the participants. Therapists who are perceived to be warm,
sincere, caring, relaxed, natural, and knowledgeable are most effective in gaining a
group's cooperation and in facilitating change.

Unlike traditionally run psychotherapy groups, pain management therapy groups
need to be focused and structured. Members need to be aware that the program is time
limited and that the raising of issues beyond the scope of pain-related concerns may not
be appropriate. When pain patients get together, there is always the risk that the discussion will degenerate into griping and grumbling. Each patient may feel that his or her
"war story" is the most tragic. Excessive complaining often leads to the group's deterioration and may cause some members to drop out. Although sharing common experiences
is important, most group members reach a point when they no longer want to hear about

problems but instead want to focus on solutions. The best therapist will allow for open sharing of information but will step in when anyone monopolizes the conversation by repeatedly recounting his or her personal problems.

GROUP FORMAT

The group format should be discussed openly at the beginning of the program and again at the start of each session. It is useful for the therapist to outline for the group what they can expect to accomplish at the session. In large groups, all members should have an opportunity to update their situation, including recent events in their lives and successes in combating their pain. Some groups agree to allow each member to speak, without questions or feedback, until everyone has spoken. Those persons who need more time to share a particularly distressing experience should be offered individual therapy. Individuals who are intolerant of other group members or who are consistently disruptive should be asked to leave.

The maximal meeting time for any group should be 1½ hours. Patients' pain usually increases when they remain stationary for a prolonged period. This exacerbation contributes to poor concentration and irritability. Patients should be told that they can stand and stretch if they need to do so.

Novel approaches to group sessions should be tried. For example, at the start of each session, members share one good and one bad thing that happened to them since the last group, without comment from others. As another option, all group members can be told to come prepared to tell a joke at the start of each session. Those who come without a joke must have two jokes ready for the next session. Also, in a large group, one patient may be appointed a "time-keeper" who ensures that all members have equal time to talk or a "record-keeper" who writes down the topics discussed and shares this information with the group at the start of the next session. The therapist may ask participants to take turns facilitating the group. A primary goal of the therapist is to promote the members' feeling of "ownership" of the group while preventing the deterioration of the meetings into "moan and groan" sessions.

FAMILY THERAPY

Chronic pain significantly impacts all members of a family. Family members need to be educated about the goals of therapy and should have an opportunity to share their concerns. Moreover, active involvement of family members helps ensure the patient's long-term success. Therefore, both patients and members of their families should be invited to attend family therapy sessions. At these sessions, the facilitator should encourage family members to ask questions about the pain management program, to discuss their concerns and expectations, and to express their feelings. Besides enhanced communication, important outcomes of these sessions are that family members learn how to help the person in pain achieve and maintain goals and that they come to understand that they are not alone in dealing with that person. It is best to schedule one family therapy session at the start and another at the end of the structured program.

COGNITIVE/BEHAVIORAL THERAPY

PRINCIPLES INFLUENCING BEHAVIOR

Five principles underlie the way in which chronic pain patients respond to treatment:

1. *Perceptions Influence Behavior.* Individuals differ in how they perceive the world. Understandably, chronic pain patients may tend to view the world in a negative light, and these negative perceptions may influence what they do. For example, patients who believe that their condition will gradually deteriorate if they are active may resist participation in an exercise program. Inaccurate information and emotional arousal can promote this type of negativity.
2. *Behavior Creates the Environment.* Individuals who act miserable and are unwilling to do things often become isolated from others. This isolation, in turn, may exacerbate feelings of depression and loneliness and may reinforce the belief that no one understands or cares what the patient is going through.
3. *Individuals Actively Assimilate Information.* In this ongoing process, pain and environmental factors continue to influence perceptions and behavior.
4. *Patients Can Learn More Adaptive Ways to Think, Feel, and Behave.* Although we tend to believe that persons with chronic pain are products of their pain and environment, it is possible to influence the way these patients think about their pain and to change their ways of coping with it.
5. *Patients Are Capable of Active Involvement in Their Own Treatment.* A strictly biomedical approach to pain control invites a passive response to treatment. However, successful rehabilitation of a patient with a chronic condition seems to be based on the patient's willingness to actively participate in getting better.

OBJECTIVES OF
COGNITIVE/BEHAVIORAL THERAPY

Cognitive/behavioral therapy has a number of objectives. The first is to help patients change their view of their problem from overwhelming to manageable. Patients who are prone to catastrophize benefit from examining the way they view their situation. What has been perceived as a hopeless condition can be reframed as a difficult yet manageable situation over which the patient can exercise some control.

The second objective is to convince patients that their treatment is relevant to their problem and that they must be actively involved both in that treatment and in their rehabilitation. They need to understand how relaxation training, cognitive restructuring, adaptive coping skills, and pacing behaviors can help decrease their pain. Patients must reorient their view away from that of passive victim to that of proactive, competent problem solver. When individuals are successful in managing painful episodes, their views change. They eventually begin to believe themselves capable of overcoming any acute flare-up of pain.

The third objective is to teach patients to monitor maladaptive thoughts and substitute positive thoughts. Persons with chronic pain are plagued, either consciously or unconsciously, by negative thoughts related to their condition. These negative thoughts have a way of perpetuating pain behaviors and feelings of hopelessness. Learning how and when to attack these negative thoughts and to substitute positive thoughts and adaptive management techniques is an important component of cognitive restructuring. Patients must be encouraged to attribute success to their own efforts; they need to feel that they are responsible for the gains they make. Finally, problems and lapses need to be discussed so that the patient will have an advance "game plan" to manage short-term setbacks.

CONTINGENCY MANAGEMENT

Most chronic pain patients need support in maintaining their gains. Important aspects of contingency management include (a) giving specific homework assignments, (b) offering appropriate examples to patients, (c) helping to organize a daily routine and schedule, (d) recruiting support from family members, (e) encouraging outside activities and involvement, (f) linking the patient to appropriate resources, (g) monitoring progress, and (h) actively following patients after treatment.

GIVE HOMEWORK ASSIGNMENTS

Before the start of each group session, patients should be assigned homework related to the topic that will be discussed. The minimum required homework may consist of reading a short chapter and writing a three-point summary of what was read. Also, any checklists, questionnaires, or surveys on the topic under discussion should be completed. The facilitator should confirm that the assignments were at least attempted. Patients who become used to completing assignments on their own initiative will likely have greater success in managing their pain after the program is over.

PROVIDE EXAMPLES
OF PROPER BEHAVIOR

Throughout the program, appropriate behavior should be modeled for group members. Techniques may include (a) describing hypothetical patients who display positive behavior, (b) pointing out individuals in the group whose behavior is positive, (c) having alumni of past programs attend sessions to discuss the benefits of their positive behavior, (d) having other professionals attend group sessions to demonstrate appropriate behavior, (e) having the facilitator demonstrate the behavior, and (f) role-playing appropriate behavior during the group sessions. Expected behavior can be modeled visually or can be described in written form or orally. Concrete examples should be given of how to adaptively cope with chronic pain. A member's achievement of a goal in the program should always be acknowledged by the group.

HELP TO CREATE A
DAILY ROUTINE

Chronic pain patients tend to let their pain dictate their activities and behavior. Patients who have external demands on their attention and time seem to adjust better to their disability. For example, patients responsible for managing small children or sticking to a regular work schedule often remain active and have set routines, if only because they feel that they have no choice. The routine should include regular times to go to bed and to get up, even if the person has had difficulty sleeping.

RECRUIT SUPPORT

Although internal and external support is an important factor in adjustment to chronic pain, such support may be hard to find. Family members and friends should be strongly encouraged to become involved in the treatment process. Likewise, patients should be encouraged to seek outside support and assistance.

ENCOURAGE RECREATIONAL
AND SOCIAL ACTIVITIES

Patients frequently state that one benefit of a pain management program is that it provides opportunities to socialize with people who understand their condition.   The regular group meeting offers a respite for some individuals. Patients who have tended to remain at home look forward to a regular time when they can leave the house, meet with others, and share their experience. This sense of belonging and routine enhances their feelings of well-being.

IDENTIFY RESOURCES

Patients with chronic pain are consumers. They need to be informed of the best resources available to aid them in the management of their pain. Apart from using the patient's handbook, *Learning to Master Your Chronic Pain* (Jamison, 1996b), they should consult libraries, bookstores, advocacy groups, pharmaceutical companies, medical centers, and computer data bases. Individuals can access important information related to their condition through the Internet and Telnet. Computer on-line services (e.g., Compuserve, America Online) sponsor open sessions through which persons with chronic pain can share information or resources. This information should be passed on to other group members.

MONITOR PROGRESS

One way patients actively participate in a pain management program is through regular monitoring of their own progress. By recording data on their pain intensity, activity levels, moods, and medications, participants gain a better understanding of their condition and of the factors that impact it. Regular monitoring takes time and effort but offers insights. Therapists should regularly inspect patients' forms and questionnaires to obtain up-to-date information and to underscore the importance of completing these documents. Filled-out forms can be collected at the end of the group session, and the information recorded can be included in discharge summaries.

STRUCTURED FOLLOW-UP

Unfortunately, the progress made over the course of a structured program is sometimes reversed within 6 months. This outcome is inevitable for some proportion of the participants in any program designed to change behavior. A way to prevent relapse is to offer a structure for follow-up, possibly including individual sessions with the group facilitator and meetings with regular support groups.

PATIENT RATING SYSTEM

It is important that patients be kept up to date about their progress. They need to know what is expected of them, how they are doing, and what to do if they are having problems. The referring physician and the insurance carrier also need to know whether a patient is improving and, if so, how much. If a patient cannot adhere to the program or is not benefiting, others need to know that, too. With a rating system like the one described next, patients can get feedback about and understand the importance of their continued participation. The result is that fewer patients leave the program prematurely.

The following modified rating system was initially created by David Schwartz, PhD (Schwartz, 1991), to provide feedback to participants in a pain management program about their progress and their perceived participation. Three aspects of each patient's progress should be rated by the staff every week:

1. *Attitude and Participation.* Actively participating in classes and groups, showing up for all activities on time, completing assignments, and exhibiting a positive attitude toward other patients are all important components of this rating.

2. *Pain Behaviors.* Behaviors like limping, rubbing, grimacing, sighing, and resting the head on the table call attention to a patient's pain, remind other patients of their own pain, and should be minimized.

3. *Compliance With Exercise and Relaxation Training.* Ratings reflect whether patients are meeting their quotas and whether they are working to improve their condition.

The therapist should review the ratings with each patient. In each of the three areas, the patient can be given a rating of 0, 1, 2, or 3. Here is what these ratings mean:

0 = *Noncompliance, Unsatisfactory.* This rating indicates total lack of involvement and/or compliance. A rating of 0 means that the patient clearly has no interest in being in the program. If a 0 rating is given, the therapist should meet with the patient to determine how to work to resolve this problem. Two 0 ratings must result in the patient's discharge from the program.

1 = *Minimal Compliance, Less Than Satisfactory.* A rating of 1 means that the patient is trying but still not making much progress. Many patients get ratings of 1 the first week, but patients who get only 1s seem not to benefit in the long run. If a patient is given a 1, a time should be set for a meeting with the therapist to come up with ideas on how to do better.

2 = *Adequate Compliance, Satisfactory.* A rating of 2 means that the patient is doing everything that is required in the program and that he or she can expect improvement if this level of participation is maintained.

3 = *Greater-Than-Required Compliance, Good/Excellent.* A rating of 3 indicates that the patient is doing more than is required and that he or she is actively participating in his or her own care, as opposed to passively complying with instructions. Patients who get 3s are the "stars" who do the best both in the program and when they go home.

The main purpose of the rating system is to help patients by making it clear what is expected of them and how they can reach their goals. If they get a rating of less than

2, they should always be told why that rating was given and what they need to do to improve it. In addition, the ratings provide a written record of each patient's effort to improve management of his or her pain.

If at any time a patient has a question or a problem with a rating or with any other aspect of the program, he or she should be able to discuss it with the therapist. However, patients should be asked not to complain about or discuss their ratings in front of other patients.

COMPLIANCE AND FOLLOW-UP

Most chronic pain patients need support after completing a pain treatment program in order to maintain their gains. Patients should be encouraged to identify and anticipate situations that place them at risk for resuming previous maladaptive behavior patterns. They should also learn to rehearse problem-solving techniques and behavioral responses that will enable them to avoid a relapse. The goals of relapse prevention are to help the patient (a) maintain a steady level of activity, emotional stability, and appropriate medication use; (b) anticipate and deal with situations that cause setbacks; and (c) acquire skills that will decrease reliance on the health care system.

Follow-up has been shown to be vital in preventing relapse. A specific, written follow-up plan should be drawn up for each patient before the end of the program. As has already been mentioned, the patient should be offered structured follow-up services, such as participation in a monthly support group session or individual sessions with the group facilitator. Individuals who are unable to complete the structured program may be invited to repeat the program another time.

A sample discharge summary for a patient who has completed a structured pain program is provided on pages 63-65. This report, which will be sent to the referring physician, reviews the patient's participation in the program and her follow-up plan.

SAMPLE DISCHARGE SUMMARY

BACKGROUND INFORMATION

Gloria Jones has been evaluated and treated at the Pain Management Center of Brigham and Women's Hospital for thoracic back pain of the T1 to T8 area. She was initially referred for treatment by Dr. John Smith and was evaluated at the Pain Management Center on 7-13-94. At that time, she was seen by Dr. Carol Kurry.

Ms. Jones was involved in a work-related incident in October 1992. She was employed as a nursing assistant at a nursing home. She recalls experiencing back pain after lifting a patient. Since that time, she has experienced mid-back pain and has been evaluated by a number of health care professionals.

Ms. Jones is currently receiving workers' compensation benefits. She is not considered a candidate for surgery. It was thought that she would benefit from the structured outpatient program for persons with chronic pain. At the time of her initial psychological evaluation, Ms. Jones described herself as very discouraged and depressed regarding her condition.

PAIN DESCRIPTION

Ms. Jones described her pain as constant in nature. The pain was located mostly at the mid-thoracic area of her back, without evidence of spreading or radiculopathy. She reported that her pain varied throughout the day, often in relation to her level of activity. At the time of her initial evaluation, she described her pain as averaging an 8 on a scale of 0 to 10.

TREATMENT GOALS

Ms. Jones attended the outpatient day program for persons with chronic pain, which began on 8-31-95 and concluded on 10-2-95. She actively participated in the program, missing only one of the sessions because of a prior commitment. At the beginning of the program, she identified some goals related to her pain. These goals included the following:

1. To gain a better understanding of her pain problems and to learn ways to deal with her pain emotionally.
2. To identify specific triggers for her pain in order to better predict fluctuations in its intensity.
3. To choose a future direction with regard to vocational retraining or productivity.
4. To gradually increase her level of activity and to engage in a regular exercise program.
5. To address weight management issues.
6. To increase her self-esteem and her sense of control over her pain.
7. To increase her ability to socialize with friends and remain active despite her discomfort.

PAIN RATINGS

Over the course of the program, Ms. Jones rated her pain twice daily, in the morning and in the afternoon. These ratings were consistently higher in the evening than in the morning; specifically, her pain ratings in the morning averaged 5 overall and varied between 3 and 9, while those in the afternoon averaged 7 and varied between 5 and 10. Although no consistent pattern was evident, her pain intensity decreased during the last 2 weeks of the program. Of particular note was a decrease in pain intensity in the afternoon, with an average rating of 5.

EXERCISE PHYSIOLOGY

Ms. Jones actively participated in the exercise component of the program. She was involved in group stretching both before and after her individual exercise session. Her cardiovascular exercises included use of the treadmill and the stationary bike. She also was involved in weight training for muscle reconditioning. Overall, her ability to participate in the cardiovascular exercises increased. She began with 10 minutes on the treadmill and progressed up to 20 minutes on the treadmill and the stationary bike. Although Ms. Jones noted an increase in pain related to her activity, she also reported an increase in endurance and stated that the stretching and exercising component of the program was beneficial to her.

MEDICATIONS

Ms. Jones has been taking Motrin 800 mg q.i.d. She also has been taking 10 mg of Elavil at night. Her over-the-counter medication includes 500 mg of Tylenol each day. One of her goals was to manage her pain without relying on medication. Elavil has been helpful in improving her sleep, and Motrin has had some ameliorating effect on her pain. In the past she has used Tylenol #3, but at this time she does not rely on any narcotic or tranquilizing medication.

BEHAVIORAL/PSYCHOLOGICAL

Ms. Jones actively participated in group therapy sessions and attended on the days that she agreed upon. She was involved in group discussion and pain management classes and seemed to benefit from interacting with the other group members. Despite some evidence of discomfort, her pain behavior and complaining were minimal. Ms. Jones stated that the information obtained through the pain program was most beneficial to her. She exhibited a noticeable difference in affect by the end of the program. She reported feeling more confident and self-assured about her condition and expressed an interest in returning to some of her previously normal daily activities. In general, Ms. Jones benefited from the education and group support offered. She described an improved sense of well-being at the conclusion of the program.

Pre- and posttreatment scores on the SCL-90, Beck Depression Questionnaire, and Coping Strategies Questionnaire showed a marked improvement in her mood and her pain beliefs. She showed less depression and greater willingness to manage her pain in active rather than passive ways.

PAIN INTERFERENCE

Ms. Jones completed a pain self-efficacy scale both at the beginning and at the end of the program. This scale measured her levels of certainty that she could perform tasks. Overall, her perception of her ability to undertake certain activities increased. In particular, she felt more certain that she could decrease her pain without relying on medication and that she could keep her pain from interfering with her sleep. She expressed greater certainty about being able to exercise at home, perform household chores, and participate in recreational activities. She also showed evidence of dealing better with emotions related to her pain. In particular, she felt more certain that she could help herself if she became discouraged or depressed and that she could deal with frustration related to controlling her pain. Overall, it appeared that Ms. Jones did show a perceptual change by the end of the program, with a better sense of control over her condition.

FOLLOW-UP PLAN

Ms. Jones addressed some specific plans for treatment after her completion of the outpatient program. The following goals were discussed:

1. *Exercise.* Ms. Jones plans to take daily walks to improve her conditioning and ensure her ability to remain active. She hopes to walk without a cane. She has recognized the importance of remaining active while learning to pace her activities. Although she plans to increase her level of activity, she recognizes that the intensity of her pain is often exacerbated by activity and has therefore been focusing on gradually increasing her activity without worsening her condition.

2. *Relaxation.* Ms. Jones participated in relaxation training and was given a relaxation cassette tape for practice purposes. She found that the relaxation training was beneficial to her. She plans to use the relaxation skills outlined in her patient's handbook along with the cassette tape. She may undertake additional sessions of thermal and EMG biofeedback as a way to decrease her sympathetic arousal and muscle spasms related to her pain.

3. *Medications.* Ms. Jones finds Elavil to be most helpful in improving her sleep and her mood. She will continue to use Motrin and over-the-counter medication. She plans to consult periodically with Dr. Kurry about medication options.

4. *Attitude and Mood.* Ms. Jones demonstrated significant changes in her affect as a result of her participation in the program. She has agreed to continue using the strategies she has learned in order to maintain a positive attitude toward the management of her pain. She feels that contact with other pain patients has been most helpful to her. She has agreed to participate in monthly group follow-up sessions offered at Brigham and Women's Hospital.

5. *Rehabilitation.* Ms. Jones plans to meet with a vocational rehabilitation counselor for a functional-capacity evaluation. She has expressed an interest in pursuing specific vocational opportunities that would move her closer to going back to work. She should enter a retraining program as soon as possible to maximize the benefits that she has obtained through the Pain Management Program.

Robert Jamison, PhD
Program Director
October 3, 1995

CHAPTER 5

Didactic Sessions

Each step of one's own is worth more than all the knowledge and insight of others.

Dorothee Soelle

PATIENT EDUCATION:
AN OVERVIEW

Most people with chronic pain have a less than adequate understanding of the nature of their painful condition and its treatment. In general, those patients who understand their condition and who apply pain management techniques when experiencing a painful episode will learn to maintain control over their pain and will have a high rate of success after completing a pain management program.

Educational group sessions are a key component in such a program. At these sessions, information can be given visually through video presentations, in writing with handouts and books, or orally in individual sessions. However, a mixed approach works best. In other words, the optimal way to educate patients is through didactic groups in which visual, written, and verbal information can be presented to many patients at once. With the patient's handbook as a guide, each group session should include a 20- to 30-minute presentation on a particular topic and a subsequent discussion. The topics covered can be chosen from the table of contents of the patient's handbook in any order that best meets the needs of the group members. Patients should be given an outline of the group sessions' topics ahead of time so that they can read the relevant chapters and complete the assignments before each session. Specific assignments should be given for each session. Again, the greater the number of sensory inputs used, the greater the chance that the information from each chapter will be remembered. Patients should first read the assigned section, write down a summary of the salient points, and then be prepared to tell other participants about what they read and wrote. The group facilitator should check to see that the assignments for each chapter are completed. Periodically, the facilitator should also ask each group member questions in order to encourage participation in the group sessions.

The educational group sessions should emphasize active learning techniques. In fact, patients should be involved in shaping these sessions by sharing their experiences; completing the surveys, checklists, and questionnaires; and contributing their ideas.

Certain "reality" themes should be highlighted throughout a structured pain program since their comprehension and acceptance are crucial to a pain management approach. These themes include the following:

1. You will most likely not be "cured."
2. You need to expect ups and downs.
3. Rarely does pain intensity remain exactly the same over time.
4. You need to have a fallback plan for those times when you have a flare-up of pain.
5. What *you* do about your pain may be as beneficial as anything that is done to or for you.
6. You need to work towards gaining control over your condition with the help of medical treatments and behavioral pain management strategies.

Information in the following sections can be adapted for use in didactic sessions in a structured pain management program.

RELAXATION TRAINING

Chronic pain patients tend to experience residual muscle tension as a function of the bracing, posturing, and emotional arousal often associated with pain. Such responses, maintained over a long period, can exacerbate pain in injured areas and increase muscular discomfort. For example, patients with low back pain or limb injuries commonly develop neck stiffness and tension-type headaches. Relaxation training can reduce pain by decreasing muscular tension, alleviating anxiety, distracting the patient from the pain, and enhancing self-efficacy in coping with pain (the belief that one can do something to produce a specific outcome). In short, this training can increase the patient's sense of control over physiological responses. In a pain management program, patients are taught a variety of relaxation strategies, including diaphragmatic breathing, progressive muscle relaxation, autogenic relaxation, imagery, and cue-controlled relaxation techniques. Biofeedback training is also commonly employed. Demonstrations of relaxation techniques are preferable to verbal explanations alone. All participants should be encouraged to practice each of the techniques during the group sessions and at home. Cassette tapes can be made for at-home practice.

Relaxation training should be presented much as a skill that comes with practice. Attempts should be made to demystify the process. Each group member should shape the relaxation techniques to meet his or her specific needs. Individuals who learn most easily through visual input may prefer relaxation techniques using imagery. Others who are more sensual and tactile may respond well to progressive muscle relaxation. Still others who are auditorily centered and rely on listening skills for optimal learning may prefer autogenic relaxation techniques.

Whether an individual continues to practice relaxation on a regular basis, the belief that something can be done to help cope with pain is maintained over time. Exposure to relaxation techniques can lead to a noticeable decrease in anxiety and a sense of confidence in dealing with severe pain.

The following are examples of relaxation strategies used for persons with chronic pain. There are a number of sources for relaxation techniques listed in the bibliography. You are encouraged to consult these texts in order to gain further knowledge of these strategies.

Progressive Muscle Relaxation

Begin by getting into as comfortable a position as you can, either seated in a chair or lying on your back. Make sure that your weight is supported completely and that your arms and legs are uncrossed. If you are seated, put both feet flat on the floor.

Now close your eyes and keep them closed. I will ask you to tense and hold and then to relax many of the muscle groups throughout the body. Let your mind focus on the different feelings that you have when you tense, hold, and then relax each muscle group.

First, concentrate on regular, smooth, easy breathing. Start by taking a deep breath, holding it, and letting it out slowly. Continue to breathe slowly and regularly while you think about relaxing. With every breath you take, imagine inhaling relaxation and exhaling tension. Inhale relaxation. Exhale tension.

We will begin with your right hand and arm. With your right hand resting on the arm of the chair, at your side, or on your lap, make a tight fist and hold it. Tense the muscles of this hand and forearm as tightly as you can, and hold it. Feel the tension as you clench your right fist. Notice how the muscles pull across the top of the hand, in the fingers, and in the upper and lower part of the forearm. Now relax. Let this arm and hand go completely limp, and pay close attention to the feeling of relaxation in these muscles. Notice how their tension gives way to complete relaxation, and focus on how completely relaxed they feel.

Now once again make a tight fist with your right hand, and hold it. Again notice how the muscles tense and pull in the arm and forearm. Relax. Feel how the relaxation flows over the hand and arm. Your hand and arm feel more and more relaxed, perhaps more deeply relaxed than ever before. Notice the difference between the tension and the relaxation.

This time tense your right biceps muscle and hold it tight. The biceps is the muscle located on top of the arm between the elbow and shoulder. You can tense it by making a muscle if you wish. Feel the tension in your biceps, and notice the contrast between that tension and the relaxation in the rest of your body. Now relax the biceps. Let your right arm fall to rest at your side. Let the relaxation flow down your arm. As your entire arm becomes more and more relaxed, just focus on this feeling of relaxation. Allow the entire right arm and hand to become deeply and totally relaxed. You may notice feelings of warmth in the fingertips as the muscles along the arm and hand become more relaxed, with feelings of looseness and heaviness along the arm.

Let's repeat the procedure now for the left arm and hand. First, make a fist with your left hand. Clench it tightly so that you can feel the muscles pull across the fingers and the upper and lower parts of the forearm. Feel the tightness and tension. Now relax. Release these muscles and let the relaxation flow in. Pay close attention to this feeling of complete relaxation as your arm and hand become more and more thoroughly and completely relaxed.

Once again, make a tight fist with your left hand, hold it, and feel the tightness and pull in the fingers and forearm. Relax. Notice how it feels as you let these muscles go completely limp and as this arm and hand continue to relax. Allow them to become as totally relaxed as your other arm and hand - thoroughly, deeply relaxed.

This time tense your left biceps muscle, and hold it tight by making a muscle. Remember, the biceps muscle is halfway between the shoulder and the elbow, on top of the arm. Feel the tension and pull. Relax. Notice how that pull of the muscle on top and under the arm goes away and is replaced by a feeling of looseness and relaxation. Just enjoy the relief and freedom from effort as both arms and hands become more and more relaxed. You may perceive sensations of warmth, heaviness, and looseness along the left arm and hand as well as the right. Allow your arms to achieve a deeper and deeper level of relaxation.

Keeping the muscles of your hands and arms relaxed, focus next on the facial muscles. First tighten the muscles in your forehead and scalp by wrinkling up your forehead and raising your eyebrows at the same time. Hold it; feel the tension. Then relax. Allow these muscles in your forehead to relax completely. Notice the difference in feeling between the relaxation, which is now taking over, and the tension, which should be going away. Allow the muscles in your forehead and scalp to become smoother and smoother.

This time squint your eyes tightly and at the same time wrinkle up your nose very tightly so that you can feel a lot of tension around your eyes and nose. Now relax. When all the muscles around your eyes and nose have relaxed completely, allow this relaxation to spread over your entire face. Keep attending to this feeling of relaxation as you let your muscles become more deeply, more thoroughly relaxed. Keep your eyelids closed very gently for the duration of this procedure. Notice and enjoy the feelings of relaxation.

This time pull back the corners of your mouth as tightly as you can. Feel the tension in the cheek and jaw muscles as you pull the corners back further and further. Relax. Notice the sensation of warmth that flows into these muscles as they become more relaxed. As you tense and relax these muscles, be sure the rest of your body remains entirely comfortable and totally relaxed as well.

This time tense your jaw muscles by biting your teeth together. Bite hard and notice the feeling of tightness in your jaw and all the way up through both temples. Now relax. Let your jaw go completely limp. Allow your teeth and your lips to part a bit and feel the surge of relief as relaxation flows back in and replaces that tension and tightness. Let your whole face become as totally relaxed as your arms and shoulders, thoroughly and deeply relaxed. Relax all these muscles further and further.

Next, push your head back as far as it will go. Notice the pressure in the back of your neck. Then relax. Let your head return to its normal position, and feel the difference. Notice how the tightness that you created in the muscles in the back of your neck gives way to a much more comfortable feeling of relaxation. Now, without creating any discomfort, bend your head forward lowering your chin as far as you can, and feel the tightness again in the back of your neck. Relax. Return your head to its normal position, and go on relaxing calmly and peacefully. You may notice an increased sensation of warmth in the muscles in the back of your neck as they relax more and more. Let your relaxation grow and deepen.

Now let's work with the shoulder muscles. With your arms still completely relaxed, raise both your shoulders up as if they were pulled up by two imaginary strings. Just lift them as high as you can, and hold the tension. Feel the pull of the large muscles across the shoulders. Then relax. Drop your shoulders as if the strings have been cut. Allow your shoulders to sag as far as they will. Experience the effortlessness and the pleasantness associated with relaxing your shoulder muscles. If your shoulders are relaxed, you should feel as if all their weight is being transferred right down through your arms and out of your body. You may notice feelings of warmth in the shoulder muscles as they become more and more relaxed. Many people find that relaxation can spread from their shoulders all the way up through the neck to the head, and all the way down both arms. Enjoy the comfortable, heavy feeling that accompanies relaxation. Let a warm flowing feeling pass over your head and down your face, across your shoulders, and down your arms to the tips of your fingers.

This time take a deep breath and hold it. Really fill your lungs. Notice how the muscles pull across your chest as you hold your breath. Now breathe out and relax. Just feel the pleasurable relief throughout your chest. Once again, take a deep breath and hold it. Again notice the increased tension and then relax. Breathe right out, relaxing and enjoying the soothing relief.

Notice how all the muscles of your body tend to become a little more relaxed when you exhale. Now breathe just a bit slower and deeper than usual. Your breathing is very easy and very rhythmical, not forced or labored in any way. Let yourself become mentally absorbed in your breathing and unaware of anything else. Just concentrate on the different sensations you experience every time you breathe in and every time you breathe out. You may find that you become a bit more relaxed with every breath you take, inhaling relaxation and exhaling tension. You may experience this increasing relaxation as a feeling of looseness: In fact, you may feel almost like a rag doll. You may also feel warmth, especially in your fingertips and toes, because more blood will reach these areas the more relaxed you become. You may experience a feeling of heaviness, as if every part of your body is being supported by whatever that part is resting on. Many people feel as if it would take a tremendous effort to get up because they feel so heavy and comfortable when they are relaxed.

Remember to be aware of your breathing. Breathe very easily, very rhythmically, a little bit more slowly than usual. Making sure that all the muscles you have already focused on remain relaxed, tighten just your stomach muscles by pulling your stomach in. Make your stomach hard, and feel what that tension is like. Now relax. Focus on the surge of relief and the complete comfort of relaxation. As your stomach muscles become completely relaxed, notice the general sense of well-being that comes with this relaxation. Allow your body to do its healing work, relaxing more and more. Continue to relax for a while, enjoying the calm and pleasant sensations of deep and total relaxation. Your arms and hands feel limp. Your shoulders are resting naturally. Your facial muscles feel relaxed and serene. Your breathing is easy and rhythmical. Very little effort is required to remain completely relaxed. You are simply allowing a natural state to develop, a natural process to occur.

Let's work next with the lower half of the body. While relaxing the rest of your body, tighten only the muscles in the upper thighs of both legs. You can do this by drawing your hips together and pressing down on your heels. Observe how it feels when you tighten both the top and the bottom thigh muscles. Now relax. Completely relax all the muscles in your legs and your stomach on up through your chest and face, arms and hands. Once again tighten the upper thigh muscles in both legs. Hold it and then relax. Feel the surge of relief as relaxation flows back in. You may feel pleasant sensations of warmth in these muscles as they become more and more thoroughly relaxed. Enjoy the good sensations that come with relaxation.

As you continue to relax all the muscles in your upper body, tense your calf muscles by pulling the ends of both feet toward your head. Keep your feet on the floor or your legs on the bed while you point your toes toward your head. Feel the tension and tightness and pull in the lower calf muscles. Now relax. Just let these muscles go. Allow the flow of relaxation to fill every muscle fiber, relaxing deeper and deeper. Now press your feet and toes downward, away from your face, so that your ankles and feet become tense. Focus on the tension in these muscles. Now relax. Relax all of the muscles in your legs and feet. Notice how the tightness that you produced in your calves gives way to a more comfortable feeling of looseness and relaxation.

Finally, push down at the same time with both your toes and heels to lift the arches in your feet. Feel the pressure, as if something were pushing up from under each arch. You will also feel a lot of pressure in your calves and shins. Now relax. Let your arches fall, and enjoy the release and freedom from effort. Go on relaxing, making quite sure that there is no tightness anywhere in your body. Just let your body totally and completely relax. Really enjoy the feeling of deep, complete, and pleasant relaxation you have created for yourself. Let yourself become even more relaxed by taking a deep breath, holding it for a few seconds, and then exhaling. As you breathe out, let your whole body relax. You may find that you become a little bit more relaxed with every breath you take. Concentrating on breathing, thinking about nothing else except breathing, allows you to relax further and further. Simply notice your breathing. Let yourself become absorbed in your breathing so that your feelings of relaxation grow stronger and stronger.

As your body relaxes more and more deeply, let your mind relax as well by thinking of a calm and peaceful place. This scene may involve being in a special spot: on the beach, in the mountains, or somewhere else. As you think about this calm and peaceful place, you may notice some particular sights, particular sounds, or smells that go with this place. Open up your senses so that you can see what you are seeing; hear what you are hearing; touch and feel what you are touching and feeling. Let your mind stay in this peaceful place. Let your body continue to relax for as long as you want to or need to. Remember to carry this feeling around with you after you open your eyes.

Autogenic Relaxation

In this session you are going to relax the involuntary muscles of your body, using a passive relaxation procedure. Get into as comfortable a position as possible. Begin by thinking about slow, regular, deep, easy breathing. Take a deep breath, hold it, and exhale any tension or tightness you may be feeling. Continue to breathe in relaxation and exhale tension. Remember that effective relaxing is a letting-go process. You can't relax if you try too hard. Instead, you need to let relaxed feelings be a part of you. If your mind starts to wander, preventing you from relaxing completely, return your attention to slow easy breathing, and concentrate on creating feelings of heaviness and warmth in your body. Allow your body's warmth and relaxation to do its healing work while your mind relaxes. With your eyes closed, continue to concentrate on deep, easy breathing throughout this session.

Now slowly, in your mind, repeat to yourself each of the phrases I say to you. Focus on each phrase as you repeat it to yourself.

I am beginning to feel calm and quiet.
I am beginning to feel quite relaxed.
My right foot feels heavy and relaxed.
My left foot feels heavy and relaxed.
My ankles, knees, and hips feel heavy, relaxed, and comfortable.
My stomach, chest, and back feel heavy and relaxed.

My neck, jaw, and forehead feel completely relaxed.
All of my muscles feel comfortable and smooth.
My right arm feels heavy and relaxed.
My left arm feels heavy and relaxed.
My right hand feels heavy and relaxed.
My left hand feels heavy and relaxed.
Both my hands feel heavy and relaxed.
My breathing is slow and regular.
I feel very quiet.
My whole body is relaxed and comfortable.
My heartbeat is calm and regular.
I can feel warmth going down into my right hand.
It is warm and relaxed.
I can feel warmth flowing down into my left hand.
It is warm and relaxed.
My hands are warm and heavy.
It would be very difficult to raise my hands at this moment.
I feel very heavy.
My breathing is slow and deep.
My breathing is getting deeper and deeper.
I am feeling calm.
My whole body is heavy, warm, and relaxed.
My whole body feels very quiet and comfortable.
My mind is still, calm, and cool.
My body is warm and relaxed.
My breathing is deeper and deeper.
I feel secure and still.
I am completely at ease.
I feel an inner peace.
I am breathing more and more deeply.

Now imagine that you are in a relaxed, comfortable, and quiet place. Remember these good, relaxed feelings as you enjoy slow, easy breathing. Continue to relax until you are ready to wake up. Then slowly stretch your fingers, toes, arms, and legs, and gradually open your eyes.

Imagery

I would like you to come with me now to a special place. This is a place of your choosing. It may be a place where you have been before, or it may be an imaginary place. It is a peaceful place where no one will bother you, where you feel safe and secure, far from any worries or concerns. Just let your imagination open up and experience this most peaceful place where you feel healed and strong. Use your imagination to see what you would see, hear what you would hear, feel what you would feel, taste and smell what you would taste and smell in this place. You will imagine yourself there without any worries or pain. You will see yourself very rested, relaxed, calm, and serene.

Let's begin by concentrating on slow, easy breathing. Allow the chair or bed to support your weight completely. Take a moment to scan your body, from the top of your head, to your toes. Notice any tension or tightness. Try to imagine that you are a hollow vessel gradually filling with a warm liquid. The liquid enters from the top of the head creating a warm, relaxed feeling throughout your scalp and face. It then flows down into your jaw and neck, down into your shoulders, and down into your arms and hands, filling up your fingers. Notice yourself beginning to feel relaxed and comfortable. Just imagine this warm, flowing liquid coating your chest and upper back. Feel warmth and relaxation flow into your waist and hips. Imagine this warm feeling flowing through your thighs, slowly filling up your legs and relaxing your knees and calves. Feel this deep warmth and relaxation throughout your feet, right down to the tips of your toes. Continue to feel sensations of warmth and heaviness while concentrating on slow, easy breathing. Gradually inhale relaxation and exhale tension and tightness. In your mind say "I am" as you inhale, and "relaxed" as you exhale. Now, with each breath, repeat to yourself, "I am relaxed."

Try to remember a favorite outdoor place where you have been by yourself. If you can remember such a place, picture in your mind how good it was to be away from everyone in this quiet, relaxed, and comfortable place. Perhaps you can recall the things that you heard, felt, or saw there. You may also remember pleasant smells. Remember the feeling you have at that time, the feeling of being at peace. Now, while you continue to relax in the chair or bed, and while you let your weight be completely supported, allow yourself to go inside your body and concentrate on smoothing every muscle group. Enjoy slow, easy breathing. Let your mind relax and your imagination open up. Follow along in your mind as you go to a very relaxing place.

Let's imagine this setting: You are on a cliff overlooking a body of water. Imagine yourself looking at the reflections in the water. Feel the breeze and the warm sun on your face. Just imagine, for a moment, what you are seeing: perhaps a few boats drifting on the water, the reflection of the sunlight on the surface of the water, and an occasional passing cloud. Imagine that you look down and see steps leading to a dock. Count these steps to yourself. You feel very comfortable, relaxed, and peaceful but also alert and awake. Imagine stepping down onto the first step, while feeling deeply relaxed. Continue down the stairs, feeling even more relaxed and comfortable. Imagine that your problems and worries are far away. Block out sounds that have nothing to do with you. Instead, enjoy the sounds of nature and the experience of being outdoors, with no worries or concerns. Now imagine yourself continuing down the stairs, all the while feeling deeply relaxed and comfortable, deeply settled and calm. Just enjoy the quiet and peaceful feelings of confidence, ease, and relaxation. Finally, imagine yourself reaching the bottom of the stairs and looking out onto the dock. Now slowly walk onto the dock. At the end of the dock, notice a small boat. Walk out and step into the boat. Notice the gentle rocking of the boat. Continue to enjoy feeling deeply and comfortably relaxed, having no worries or concerns, and taking in all the sensations of being outside.

Set the boat free to drift, or just be in the boat while it remains tied to the dock, rocking back and forth, back and forth. You may feel a bit drowsy - almost as if you could go to sleep. Be aware of feeling very deeply relaxed, of having no worries. Imagine what you are seeing around you, what you are hearing, what you are smelling and touching. Now, while you continue to enjoy these sensations, drift back to the dock and slowly step out of the boat. Look around while you take a deep breath. Enjoy being outside on a beautiful day. Feel the cool breeze; look at the water; experience the comfort of being alone and quiet, feeling restful and at peace.

As you turn around and look at the steps, be aware of how relaxed and calm you feel. Step up onto the first step, feeling light and very relaxed. Slowly step up onto the next step, noticing how relaxed you continue to feel. Now continue climbing the steps feeling very comfortable, relaxed, and settled. Eventually you come to the place where you started; you turn around and notice everything around you: the water, the boats, the sky, and the clouds. Enjoy this moment still free of worries and concerns. Notice that your breathing is easy; notice that your mind feels relaxed and worry-free. You are glad for this moment. You are glad to be alive. You feel relaxed and safe, confident and strong.

You may recall a time when you first woke up in the morning after a sound sleep and became aware of light. You kept your eyes closed but knew that you were awake; feeling relaxed, comfortable, and at ease. In a moment you will count down from 5 to 1, noticing the feeling of deep relaxation, while you imagine waking up. Slowly count from 5 to 1. Then gradually open your eyes, stretch your fingers and toes, and be aware of the feelings of deep relaxation that have stayed with you.

EXERCISE

Most chronic pain patients are physically deconditioned because of a reluctance to exercise and a perceived need to protect themselves from additional physical injury. Some patients have been medically advised to restrict their activity when their pain increases. Patients should be educated on the importance of exercise in the treatment of chronic pain. The emphasis should be on stretching, cardiovascular exercise, and weight training. Each patient should be asked to keep track of all exercises in an exercise record (see pages 105-106).* It is important to set an exercise quota to be met every week. The exercise plan is initially determined by the patient and is reviewed and supervised by a physical therapist or exercise physiologist. Because patients tend to comply well with exercise in a group setting, offering a time for group members to exercise together can be beneficial, especially to those who are anxious about worsening their condition. Patients should be encouraged to loosen up by stretching before and after each exercise session. After warm-up stretches, all participants should be given an opportunity to work on their individual exercise quota either with individual exercise equipment or by walking.

---

*Note: The Exercise Record (p. 106), Medication Record (p. 110), Sleep Diary (p. 114), SOLVE-Problems Worksheet (pp. 117-118), and Daily Food Diary (p. 120) are also reproduced in a smaller format in the patient's handbook, *Learning to Master Your Chronic Pain*. If you need additional copies of these forms for use with your patients, they may be reproduced.

In any exercise program, chronic pain patients are bound to encounter some disappointments and perceived failures. Patients may at first make excellent gains, only to experience a later flare-up. These setbacks should be anticipated to avoid excessive disappointment. Behavioral research suggests that compliance with exercise is best in a structured setting where each person is monitored and encouraged about his or her accomplishments. Unfortunately, follow-up 6 months after the conclusion of a treatment program indicates that persons with chronic pain tend not to continue with a regular exercise regimen. Ways to encourage exercise, such as organizing an exercise group with other patients, joining a health club, or combining exercise with another everyday activity, should be explored.

STRETCHING

Before beginning group exercise, each patient should meet with a physiatrist, physical therapist, or exercise physiologist to tailor the exercises appropriately. Particular caution should be used in situations where stretching exercises may aggravate pain. Stretching illustrations are included in *Learning to Master Your Chronic Pain* (Jamison, 1996b), which will hereafter be referred to in this book as the patient's handbook.

It is helpful to do group stretches together, with a leader demonstrating the techniques. Exercises should be done in a room that has ample space for lying on the floor and moving around. A facility with a bar attached to the wall for use with calf stretches is ideal. Mirrors may make some patients feel self-conscious. Patients should be told ahead of time that the exercise component of the pain management program is designed to increase flexibility and strength and that all patients - no matter what their current weight and condition - can benefit. In other words, patients should be put at ease and encouraged not to feel self-conscious. Toward the end of the program, some group members may want to lead the stretches.

Various stretch bands can be used in group stretching sessions; these bands can be taken home for practice. Music may also be an enjoyable accompaniment to stretching activities.

CARDIOVASCULAR EXERCISE

The cardiovascular component of the exercise program is designed to increase endurance and self-confidence and should be individualized for each patient. Patients are encouraged to begin cautiously, doing only a little cardiovascular exercise during the first week (e.g., 10 minutes of walking, 5 minutes on a treadmill, or 5 minutes on a stationary bike once or twice a day). If some patients push themselves too far, the consequences may negatively affect their belief that exercise is beneficial. It is most important to avoid overexertion. A common scenario is for a patient to feel good on the first day of exercise and then to report a significant increase in pain and discomfort on the following day.

Patients are encouraged to try out different exercises in order to find out which is best for them and to minimize any exacerbation of their pain. Walking may have the same aerobic benefit as using exercise equipment.

Patients are first asked to establish a comfortable rate and duration of exercise and to monitor this activity for 1 week. During this baseline period a minimum exercise quota can be set. Ideally, this quota will gradually be increased to 10 to 20 minutes of cardio-vascular exercise 3 days a week.

WEIGHT TRAINING

Some patients may be interested in weight training using Nautilus-type equipment. This course should be pursued cautiously with close monitoring by the physical therapist and exercise therapist. Certain exercises designed to strengthen muscles in the upper and lower portion of the body may prove beneficial; however, many types of weight-lifting exercises may only exacerbate pain. In other cases, although weight training may not lessen pain intensity, it may help to improve the patient's self-confidence and belief in his or her ability to meet physical challenges.

ROLE OF MEDICATION

The main difference between man and animals is the desire to take medicine.

Sir William Osler

The role of medications for chronic pain is an important topic for discussion in the didactic sessions. The chapter on the role of medication in chronic pain in the patient's handbook is meant to be a brief introduction to this topic; more detailed information should be presented during these discussions. Medication records need to be reviewed and questions about their medications answered.

Patients often know little about the medications that they take and are frequently confused about commonly used terms such as *tolerance*, *physical dependence*, and *addiction*. Many patients are uninformed about the different categories of medications prescribed for pain or are uncertain where their medications fit into these categories. Many have questions regarding interactions with other medications and possible adverse effects. Moreover, patients often lack information about the risks and benefits of taking medications over a long period.

In discussions of the role of medication in the treatment of chronic pain, it is most helpful to have a physician who can cover the general topic and then focus on individual medications. The group's facilitator must also be familiar with medications frequently prescribed for chronic pain.

DEFINITION OF TERMS

Terms associated with the use of medication for chronic pain should be defined. It is important to emphasize that physical dependence on medication is not synonymous with addiction. Physical dependence is a physiologic state that is manifested by somatic symptoms (e.g., fatigue, increased pain, nausea, vomiting) and that accompanies the discontinuation of therapy with some drugs (especially opioids).

The World Health Organization defines addiction as

> a state, psychic and sometimes also physical, resulting from the interactions between a living organism and a drug, characterized by behavioral and other responses that always include a compulsion to take the drug on a continuous or periodic basis to experience its psychic effects, and sometimes to avoid the discomfort of its absence. Tolerance may or may not be present. (World Health Organization, 1986, p. 4)

Persons who are addicted to a drug have a compulsion to take it because of its euphoric effects. They also tend to display antisocial behavior in an attempt to get a drug. Evidence exists that persons with chronic pain develop tolerance and physical dependence when taking opioid medication but do not necessarily become addicted.

CATEGORIES OF MEDICATION

Medications for chronic pain patients fall into five groups: (a) nonsteroidal anti-inflammatories, (b) opioid analgesics, (c) antidepressants, (d) tranquilizers and sedatives, and (e) other adjuvant medications.

Nonsteroidal Anti-Inflammatory Drugs (NSAIDs). NSAIDs work on the peripheral level of the body by inhibiting the synthesis of prostaglandins, which contributes to pain. These drugs are useful for the treatment of arthritic pain, as well as dental pain, back pain, headaches, and postoperative pain. NSAIDs differ from one another with respect to the duration and action. Patients may benefit from one NSAID and not from another. This type of medication is often prescribed first for persistent pain. NSAIDs can be combined with other medications for enhanced benefit.

The adverse effects of the chronic use of NSAIDs include gastrointestinal upset (with ulceration and bleeding in some cases), increased bleeding time, and liver disease. These agents exhibit a "ceiling effect:" a maximal analgesic impact that cannot be increased by the administration of higher doses. Tolerance to these medications does not develop. NSAIDs pose certain risks to elderly patients and to patients with a history of heart failure, renal insufficiency, poor circulation, and ongoing diuretic therapy.

Opioid Medications. Opioids (also known as narcotics) work mostly within and around the central nervous system by binding to various opioid receptors. Unlike

NSAIDs, opioids do not exhibit a ceiling effect and are limited in their impact only by their adverse effects. Weak opioids in the usual doses are often no more effective than NSAIDs. Opioids are classified as agonists, partial agonists, and mixed agonist-antagonists. Patients are often given a starting dose, which is then increased gradually. Adverse effects (including sedation, grogginess, dizziness, nausea, vomiting, and constipation) often lessen with time, as do the analgesic effects. Morphine is the standard of comparison for the strong opioids and codeine for the weak opioids.

Considerable controversy exists about the use of opioid analgesics for the treatment of chronic nonmalignant pain. Much of this controversy is related to concerns about efficacy, adverse effects, tolerance, and addiction. Some clinicians and researchers believe that long-term opioid use contributes to psychological distress, poor outcome, impaired cognition, and excessive reliance on the health care system. Others argue that chronic opioid therapy for nonmalignant pain is sometimes appropriate; they cite the relatively low incidence of abuse and addiction among patients given opioids and report that tolerance does not develop in many patients with stable pain pathophysiology.

Current guidelines suggest that the administration of opioids should be considered only after all other reasonable attempts at analgesia have failed. Opioid therapy is contraindicated by a history of substance abuse, a major psychiatric diagnosis, the seeking of drugs from more than one physician, uncontrolled dose escalation, and/or evidence of lack of compliance. Patients with significant adverse reactions to low-dose opioid therapy are also poor candidates for such treatments. Other "red flags" include extremely high ratings of pain intensity and emotional distress, a perceived inability to cope, use of multiple pain descriptors, a perceived low level of social support, pain at multiple sites, a poor employment history, and long-term reliance on health care professionals. The decision to use opioid therapy often rests on clinical judgment and treatment orientation. The actual significance of the factors just discussed is speculative at best, and - until controlled clinical trials are conducted - they cannot be considered reliable contraindications of chronic opioid therapy for nonmalignant pain.

Patients prescribed chronic opioid therapy should take their medication on a regular basis rather than on an as-needed schedule; patients can omit a dose during the times when their pain is not severe. For chronic use, a long-acting opioid (e.g., methadone) is preferable to a short-acting medication (e.g., Percocet). Patients discontinuing opioid medication can experience withdrawal effects resembling severe flu. Tolerance is common among patients who have taken opioids for a long period of time. Patients who rapidly develop tolerance to medication are not considered good candidates for opioid therapy. A sample of an opioid therapy contract is included on page 107.

Antidepressants. Antidepressant medication (e.g., amitriptyline) is commonly prescribed for patients in chronic pain. Some antidepressants contribute to brain levels of serotonin, which is known to reduce pain transmission. The doses used typically are lower than those given to persons treated for depression. These drugs have a number of adverse effects but are generally considered safe for long-term use. The side effects may include dry mouth, urinary retention, sedation, low blood pressure upon standing up suddenly, constipation, blurred vision, and weight gain. Antidepressant medication is most helpful in cases including neuropathic pain or burning pain. Because of their sedating qualities, antidepressants can also alleviate sleep problems.

Tranquilizers and Sedatives. Major tranquilizers were initially developed to help calm patients with severe mental illness. They have an antipsychotic effect that results in improved thinking in these cases. Chronic use of tranquilizers and sedatives by chronic pain patients is not recommended. Major tranquilizers (e.g., Thorazine) have been used for treating anxiety and nausea; however, they do not significantly control pain and can produce a state of extreme sedation, low blood pressure, and respiratory depression. Other adverse effects include dry mouth and urinary retention.

Minor tranquilizers (e.g., Valium) - known as benzodiazepines - have been used to aid sleep and to decrease muscle spasms and anxiety. These agents can decrease pain, possibly because they relax the whole body. They can be helpful for short-term use, but their extended use may contribute to abnormal sleep patterns and depression (to which many chronic pain patients are prone) as well as psychological and physical dependence. Other side effects include drowsiness, decreased memory, impaired thinking, and fatigue. Muscle relaxants (e.g., Flexeril) help to decrease muscle spasms associated with chronic pain; they also have a sedative effect, and after long-term use patients become dependent on them without experiencing pain relief.

Other Adjuvant Medications. A number of other adjuvant medications are prescribed for chronic pain. These include anticonvulsants (e.g., Tegretol), corticosteroids, (e.g., Prednisone), barbiturates (e.g., Phenobarbital), antihistamines (e.g., Vistaril), psycho-stimulants (e.g., Ritalin), and oral local anesthetics (e.g., Mexitil).

Anticonvulsants are helpful in the treatment of shooting neural pain (which may also be described as lancinating, piercing, or intermittent). These drugs were originally developed to prevent epileptic seizures. They calm the electroactivity of the nerves without overly sedating the individual. The adverse effects of these medications can include liver and bone marrow damage. Anticonvulsants can also contribute to mental cloudiness, slurred speech, dizziness, and poor muscle coordination. However, under proper supervision, chronic pain patients have taken anticonvulsants for long periods without complications.

No research findings suggest that the use of other adjuvant medications for extended periods is appropriate for persons with chronic pain. However, some physicians prescribe these agents anyway to see if they are beneficial. Corticosteroids alleviate severe inflammation but have considerable adverse effects that limit their chronic use.

Antihistamines alleviate sleep problems. Some individuals reportedly benefit from psychostimulants and oral anesthetics although long-term benefits are generally minimal.

MONITORING OF MEDICATIONS

Medication records kept by patients should include the name of each medication, the date and time when it is taken, and the dosage. Before entering a structured program, the patients should monitor their medication for 1 week. The medication record should be completed at the end of the program to assess changes. This information is helpful in documenting the effect of the program on medication use and in increasing the patient's awareness of his or her own patterns of medication use (see Sample Medication Record on pp. 109-110).

The scales created to help clinicians quantify the use of medication regimens include the Medication Quantification Scale (MQS; Steedman et al., 1992). With the MQS, scores can be calculated on the basis of weighted values for medication classes (nonprescription medication = 1; NSAIDs = 2; antidepressants = 2; muscle relaxants = 3; benzodiazepines = 4; weak opioids = 4; barbiturates/sedatives = 5; and strong opioids = 6) and dosage levels (nonopioid dosage based on therapeutic level, opioid dosage based on milligram morphine equivalent). The scores can be summed to obtain a quantitative index of total medication use.

Commercial devices have also been developed to monitor compliance with medication. One such device is the Medication Event Monitoring System (MEMS; Aprex Corporation), in which the date and time are recorded whenever a container of medication is opened. There is, however, no foolproof way to accurately monitor compliance with treatment. Ultimately, patients must recognize their responsibility for their own compliance and the importance of compliance to their well-being.

Monitoring Adverse Effects. Side effects should be monitored regularly during treatment for chronic pain. Periodic monitoring of adverse effects by means of a checklist can provide relatively objective data for use in the assessment of treatment. Such a checklist may include drowsiness, dizziness, impaired coordination, irritability, depression, headache, memory lapse, dry mouth, visual distortions, nausea, vomiting, sweating, constipation, heart palpitations, itching, breathing problems, nightmares, and difficulty in urinating. Each of these symptoms can be rated on a scale from 0 (absent) to 3 (severe) (see Side Effects Checklist, p. 111). Although patients frequently report adverse effects of medication during the initial stage of treatment, many of these reactions diminish over time.

The appendix on pages 153-165 lists medications commonly prescribed for patients with chronic pain. These tables include generic names, brand names, standard dosages, and other relevant information.

STRESS AND PAIN MANAGEMENT

Stress management is a popular topic in business and work environments and is an important area of discussion in a program for persons with chronic pain. Patients often report being stressed by their pain and cite this stress as the cause of many problems.

Hans Selye, MD (Selye, 1956, 1975), spent much of his career examining human reactions to stress, which he defined as a "nonspecific response of the body to a demand." He identified physiologic phenomena that are often documented when an individual is experiencing extreme emotional arousal. These phenomena include increases in muscle tension, heart rate, respiration, adrenal gland secretion, and blood pressure; constriction of blood vessels in the extremities; difficulty with concentration and memory; and fluctuations in mood.

Dr. Selye defined a stressor as a stimulus (or cause) and a stress response as the emotional and physical reaction to that stimulus (or effect). Chronic pain is both a stressor and a stress response. Pain is emotionally arousing, and emotional arousal contributes to greater pain. Decreased arousal, in the form of relaxation, has a calming effect on pain that can help to break the cycle.

Although in most people's minds stress has negative connotations, it can in fact be either good or bad. An illustration of "good stress," that can be presented to a pain management group, is a skydiver who is poised to leap from an airplane. She will experience the physiological and emotional arousal that comes with preparation for a stressful event. Her muscles will be tense, her heart rate rapid, her breathing shallow, and her mind occupied by thoughts of what she should do. Her hands and feet will be cool because, under stressful conditions, her blood vessels will be constricted. Adrenaline levels in her blood will rise and various hormonal changes will take place. This stress reaction is important in her ability to land safely and escape harm.

However, this same reaction is injurious if it continues for days or weeks. Although some emotional arousal is needed for maximal productivity, a prolonged stress response has an adverse effect on the body - similar to the damage to the car that would result if the driver stepped on the gas and the brake simultaneously and raced the engine for a long time. Persons with chronic pain are highly susceptible to chronic arousal because of the persistent nature of their condition. Their muscles remain tense around the pain site, they have anxiety reactions when their pain flares up, and they frequently worry about their situation. These patients need to learn to manage both the stressors and their responses to them.

Figure 5.1 (p. 84) illustrates this point. It represents a beaker of water with a cap on it that is set on a burner. The low water level before warming represents a stable level of emotion. The flame represents external stress, while the cap on the beaker represents the control and suppression of physical and emotional reactions. Over time, pressure builds up in the beaker and the water level rises. Under stress the ability to reason objec-

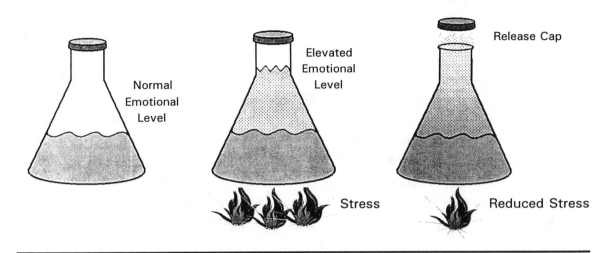

Figure 5.1. Stress Management Illustration.

tively decreases, and control of the emotions becomes difficult. The risk of prolonged stress is that the beaker will eventually crack or even explode. There are two ways to prevent this outcome: decreasing the heat (dealing with the stressor) and/or slowly letting the pressure off (dealing with the stress response). In the illustration, the pressure can be eliminated by lowering and finally extinguishing the flame or by releasing the cap (or attaching a runoff valve). For patients with chronic pain, pressure may be reduced by saying no to outside demands, pacing daily activities, using distraction and relaxation strategies, and learning to express frustration in an acceptable manner.

Another concept related to stress management is the notion of distinguishing between what one can and cannot control and then letting go of the things that are out of one's control. For example, chronic pain has a limiting effect. Individuals who are used to being very active and managing their own affairs find that they are limited by their pain. They can no longer do things for others or for themselves as they have in the past. Group members need to identify those things that they can control and know what is out of their control. In addition, many patients are concerned that other people do not understand what they are going through. Although they can try to explain their experience to others, most people still will not grasp the extent of the effect of chronic pain. Patients need to realize that this situation is out of their control. Relentless worry about not being understood by family members or friends is futile. If patients simply acknowledge their own concern about how others feel about them while recognizing that they have little control over this situation, their emotional stress and worry may be alleviated. It is also helpful for patients to share their concerns with other group members, who may be able to help them break the cycle of "bad" stress listed in the patient's handbook (pp. 69-73). Give some examples, and then ask for suggestions from group members. Have each participant identify a stressful event that has taken place within the past few weeks; then use the stress management checklist (p. 75) to assess how the individual managed that event. Focus attention on those items that were circled "no." Talk about which items could be described as stressors and which as stress responses.

SLEEP DISTURBANCES

One of the most common complaints of persons with chronic pain is an inability to sleep. These patients not only have trouble getting to sleep but also tend to wake up periodically throughout the night for various reasons (e.g., because they turn over onto a painful area or because they become stiff after remaining stationary for a long time). Never feeling completely rested has a negative influence on mood and often contributes to the exacerbation of pain.

Patients frequently have misconceptions about sleep. For instance, people think they should have 7 or 8 hours of sleep. Contrary to what many believe, however, moderate sleep loss does not necessarily affect performance during the next day, and we can often manage with less sleep than we think. The most important principle to apply to sleep disturbances is to stop *trying* to sleep. Rather than tossing and turning in bed all night worrying about not getting to sleep, the focus must be on creating conditions in which sleep will come naturally.

Each patient should complete the sleep diary in the patient's handbook before the group session on sleep-related problems in order to identify his or her individual sleep patterns. It is important to discuss sleep stages, rapid eye movement (REM) sleep, and circadian rhythm with the group. The sleep improvement strategies in the patient's handbook should be discussed, and participants should be encouraged to try each one. (See Sample Sleep Diary on pp. 113-114)

Many chronic pain patients have been prescribed medications (e.g., tricyclic antidepressants or sedatives) to improve their sleep and alleviate their pain. It is helpful to discuss how these medications work to improve sleep and to distinguish between those on which patients can become dependent (e.g., Halcion) and those which are sedating but seem not to carry a risk of physical dependence (e.g., Elavil).

Some chronic pain patients worry about using any medication to help them get to sleep. They need to be reassured that, on occasion, sleeping medication can be helpful. Patients who remain apprehensive may, for example, decide to take one pill every 3 days. This regimen will ensure that they will get some sleep even if their sleeplessness prevails.

In addition, behavioral techniques, such as those listed in the patient's handbook, are effective in improving sleep if used on a regular basis. Chronic pain patients may initially find these techniques frustrating, but, with practice, their sleep will improve. Behavioral techniques are not always helpful during a crisis but can be used to gradually improve the duration and frequency of sleep. Chronic pain patients need to recognize that during a painful episode they almost inevitably will have greater difficulty in getting to sleep at night. A fallback plan for those times should be devised so that patients do not become inordinately distressed over their lack of sleep.

Pain patients can be helped simply by knowing that chronic sleep disturbances are common. Expressing their concerns in a group setting can be comforting and reassuring. Group members can share tips on improving sleep. The facilitator should be aware of other problems that may contribute to sleep disturbances, such as chronic alcohol abuse, sleep apnea, restless leg syndrome, and long-standing psychological problems.

COMFORT MEASURES

For all the happiness mankind can gain
It is not in pleasure but in rest from pain.
John Dryden

Patients with chronic pain should be informed consumers who know what treatments are available and the positive and negative aspects of each. A session should be devoted to reviewing all of the current treatments. Many patients will state that they have already tried most of these treatments, with limited success. The goal of the review is not to encourage a fresh trial of those interventions but rather to help group members understand the options and participate in decisions about what is best for them. Inviting practitioners from other disciplines to come to this session and explain the different interventions would be helpful.

The difference between passive treatments and active treatments should be highlighted. Passive treatments are regimens used to relieve pain that are either given by someone else or self-administered. They do not require practice or active participation - hence the designation "passive." Table 5.1 (pp. 87-88) lists some current passive treatments for pain in the order of their perceived invasiveness. Most of the strategies outlined in the patient's handbook are active treatments.

ASSERTIVENESS TRAINING

A primary complaint of persons with chronic pain is that they are limited in function and activity. Tasks that were easy for them in the past may now be very difficult because of the nature of their pain. Patients commonly complain that it takes much more time to complete a task and that there are some activities in which they can no longer participate. Their consequent need for assistance from others contributes to feelings of guilt, anger, and frustration. Some patients keep their needs to themselves and

TABLE 5.1: PASSIVE TREATMENTS OF CHRONIC PAIN

Treatment	Description	Positive Aspects	Negative Aspects
Heat and cold	Hot packs or ice	Good temporary relief	Risk of burning or freezing skin
Massage	Performed by a massage therapist	Good short-term benefit	No insurance coverage
Ultrasound	Deep-heat treatment performed by a physical therapist	Temporary benefit in relaxing muscles	Benefits short-lived
Transcutaneous electrical nerve stimulation (TENS)	Portable unit with electrodes using a 9-volt battery; stimulates nerve endings to block the pain signal	Minimal adverse effects; can be adjusted by patient and used at home	Effectiveness is lost over time; the unit can be difficult to put on alone
Hypnosis	Relaxation induction technique with suggestions performed by a hypnotist	Pain relief and decreased anxiety for some suggestible patients	Induction technique not helpful for some patients; effects sometimes short-lived
Acupuncture	Thin needles placed by an acupuncturist	Adequate pain relief in some cases; potential relaxing effect	Often not covered by insurance; some risks if not performed properly
Magnotherapy	High-powered magnets placed over pain sites	Noninvasive, with pain relief in some cases	Efficacy not proven
Nerve blocks	Injections of local anesthetic, with or without steroid, often by an anesthesiologist	Proven short-term effect; long-term help for some individuals	Injections sometimes painful; complications possible
Medications	Various medications prescribed for chronic pain (see Appendix, pp. 153-165)	May decrease pain and improve sleep, function, and mood	Have different short- and long-term adverse effects; may lead to physical and/or psychological dependence

Treatment	Description	Positive Aspects	Negative Aspects
Implantable devices	Spinal cord stimulator, with electrode lead inserted into the spine and connected to a battery-powered receiver; morphine pump, an implanted chamber sending the drug through a catheter to the pain site	Both units helpful in relieving pain	Both units expensive; periodic service is needed; long-term efficacy not determined
Neurosurgical treatments	Nerves surgically severed, removed, or ablated by a neurosurgeon	Pain relief	Considerable residual effects and recurrence of pain possible

push themselves beyond their limits in order to avoid asking for help. Unfortunately, the result is often further pain and frustration. Other patients find themselves becoming very irritable and getting into frequent arguments with family members and friends.

Assertiveness training helps persons with chronic pain to identify their most effective communication style and to use it to their best advantage. Patients need to realize they are their own best advocates; no one else knows how their pain affects them. They need to stand up for themselves and convey information about their pain in as objective a manner as possible without infringing on the rights of others.

The facilitator can present frequently encountered scenarios to group members and can help each individual understand the way he or she reacts in difficult situations. The scenarios may be read aloud, with members writing their responses to each in the handbook. After everyone has had a chance to write down a response, the situations can be discussed. The following are sample scenarios.

What do you do under the following circumstances?

1. You are committed to attend a social event, but your pain tells you that you should stay home. If you don't go, you will let down your family and friends. If you do go, you will suffer for the next 2 days.
2. You are having a particularly bad day with your pain. While you are patiently waiting in line at a store, another customer cuts in line ahead of you.
3. Despite your pain, you agree to go to a restaurant for dinner. You order your favorite meal, but when it arrives you discover that it is barely warm.
4. Your physical therapist insists on certain exercises that dramatically increase your pain. She believes that they help you, but you believe that the exercises cause more harm than good.

5. You have some chores at home that require reaching and bending and that you know will increase your pain. A family member innocently points out that you have not done the chores yet.

As group members discuss each situation, it is important to understand how each individual communicates with the others about his or her pain. For example, one member may state, "I have always been quiet. I keep my feelings to myself, and I can't change now." It is helpful to point out that although personality styles are different, assertiveness is a behavior that can be learned. Patients who are neither aggressive nor overly passive but who can express their feelings and explain their restrictions in an open, objective manner tend to manage better with their pain. This topic may also be discussed in family meetings and coincides with the chapters on problem solving and stress management in the patient's handbook.

DEPRESSION, PAIN, AND POSITIVE THINKING

Part of every misery is the fact that you don't merely suffer but have to keep on thinking about the fact that you suffer. I not only live each endless day in grief, but live each day thinking about living each day in grief.

C. S. Lewis

Chronic pain patients are subject to depression and negative thinking, and they need to gain insight into managing their moods. The chapters on pain and positive thinking and on pain and depression in the patient's handbook can be presented either together or separately. The primary goal of these chapters is to help patients realize that their perception of events (rather than just the events themselves) can influence their reaction. In the course of discussions on these topics, it is important to explain the notions of "inner self" and "self-talk."

NEGATIVE THINKING

Patients are quick to recognize that during a flare-up they repeat negative self-statements. Statements patients make in the group can be used to illustrate this point. The facilitator should ask the members what their worst fears or worries are during a painful flare-up. Often patients have negative thoughts like "My pain is getting worse," "I can't deal with this pain any longer," and "I can't go on like this." The diagram in Chapter 10 (p. 104) of the patient's handbook should help patients understand that self-talk contributes to emotional reactions. This diagram illustrates the theory behind rational-emotive therapy. Patients who develop a "new" pain often worry about their condition. They may have negative, irrational thoughts about the pain that they neither test nor challenge (e.g., "I have a rare disease that the doctors cannot detect, and I will surely die" or "This pain means that I will have to have my leg amputated"). A patient's rational challenging of negative thoughts can help reduce the emotional reaction to pain. In establishing this point, it is helpful to use a specific situation presented by a group member as an illustration.

Patients should be asked to complete the Inventory of Negative Thoughts in Response to Pain (INTRP; pp. 107-108 of the patient's handbook) as part of their home-work assignment (Gil et al., 1990). The INTRP is scored by each individual as follows: never = 0, seldom = 1, sometimes = 2, often = 3, and always = 4. A total score and three subscale scores are then calculated. The first subscale is "Negative Self-Statements," which entails the sum of the ratings for items 1, 5, 6, 10, 11, 12, 14, 16, 17, 19, and 21 divided by 11. The second, "Negative Social Cognitions" consists of the sum of the ratings for items 2, 4, 7, 8, 15, 18, and 20 divided by 7. The subscale for "Self-Blame" is scored by summing the ratings for items 3, 9, and 13 and dividing the result by 3. The total score is calculated as the total number of items endorsed, regardless of rating (i.e., any rating > 0). The average frequency is the sum of all ratings for all endorsed items divided by the number of items. Patients can complete this scale at home and score it with the group. Patients who endorse more than 13 negative thoughts, regardless of the rating assigned, are considered to exhibit a higher-than-average level of endorsement of negative thoughts. Patients who have an average frequency rating of > 2.0 are consid-ered to have a higher-than-average tendency toward recurrent negative thoughts. This information helps patients assess their propensity to have recurrent negative thoughts during a flare-up of pain. This exercise helps patients realize that positive thinking im-proves coping.

Two terms that should be discussed during the presentation of this topic are "catastrophizing" and "absolutizing." Catastrophizing is a tendency to dwell on the nega-tive aspects of any experience and to contemplate the worst possible scenario associated with that experience, whereas absolutizing is a tendency to interpret any event in black-and-white terms. Patients need to realize that most situations are neither all bad nor all good and that overreacting to any new situation tends to make it worse. In other words, it is best to respond to any new condition like a dimmer (with a slow, gradual reaction) rather than a light switch (either on or off).

An outline in Chapter 10 (pp. 103-105) in the patient's handbook illustrates ways to overcome irrational thoughts. Each patient should be asked to identify one recurrent pain-related thought and to answer the questions listed on page 105 of the handbook. In addition, the group should come up with examples of positive thoughts that can be substi-tuted for negative thoughts.

DEPRESSION

It is natural for chronic pain patients to be depressed at times because of their pain. If participants in a pain management program are asked to describe someone who is depressed, they may characterize that person as one who looks tired, sad, or uncomfortable; has sleep and appetite problems; has a hard time remembering things; has no sex drive; and contemplates suicide. This description also applies to someone who is in pain. Making this connection helps participants realize that pain and depression are related and that other people may have difficulty telling the difference.

Differences between exogenous and endogenous depression should be discussed in the group session. Participants in pain programs often identify differences between depression associated with a "chemical imbalance" and depression due to stressful life events. Patients need to talk about these differences and to realize that pain can cause depression that has both an endogenous and an exogenous component; that is, pain is both an internal, physiological experience and a highly stressful event with many implications for lifestyle. Other topics for discussion include the usefulness of antidepressant medications for persons experiencing chronic pain and the stigma associated with having a mood disorder associated with pain. A related point is that many individuals (including health care professionals) believe that an underlying mood disorder actually accounts for a patient's chronic pain.

Treatments for depression should be reviewed with an emphasis on the roles of medications, cognitive therapy, interpersonal therapy, exercise, and relaxation. It is helpful for patients to complete a depression inventory - either the Beck Depression Inventory (BDI; Beck & Steer, 1987) or the Center for Epidemiological Studies-Depression Scale (CES-D; Radloff, 1977). Patients who score higher than 13 on the BDI or higher than 15 on the CES-D are classified as mildly to moderately depressed. It should be pointed out that many of the items that contribute to elevated depression scores reflect somatic complaints (e.g., loss of sexual interest) rather than cognitive concerns (e.g., feelings of hopelessness about the future). These somatic complaints are typically endorsed by persons with persistent pain.

PROBLEM SOLVING

The art of life is the art of avoiding pain; and he is the best pilot, who steers clearest of the rocks and shoals with which it is beset.

Thomas Jefferson

Everyone has a capacity to solve problems. However, individuals with chronic pain often lack confidence in their ability to find solutions to problems associated with their condition. Chronic pain contributes to feelings of inadequacy about performing even the simplest of tasks including solving problems. In a pain management program patients can learn problem-solving techniques applicable to their situation. They can use the SOLVE-Problems Worksheet to derive solutions (see example on pages 115-116). This was adapted from the *Self-Management Training Program for Chronic Headache: Patient Manual--Volume II* (in press) created by Donald Penzien, PhD and Jeanette Rains, PhD. The mnemonic for this technique is: S (state the problem), O (outline the problem), L (list possible solutions), V (view the consequences), and E (execute the solution).

To help group members gain a thorough understanding of this problem-solving technique, a review of the text can be preceded by an assignment in which each patient first identifies a particular problem associated with pain. It is best to tackle problems that are specific and easily stated (e.g., "I can't unload the dishwasher without extreme pain") rather than nonspecific (e.g., "I am useless around the house"). Participants are asked to read the section on problem solving and to come to the group session with their identified problem so that the group can act as a "brain trust" in coming up with solutions for that problem. Before the participants' problems are examined, it is helpful to review with them an example like the one presented at the end of this chapter. Then the plan below can be followed:

Draw an outline of the SOLVE-Problems Worksheet on a drawing board for display during the group session. Ask group members what they know about left- and right-brain function. The left side of the brain is characterized by objectivity and critical thinking; individuals in whom this side of the brain is dominant tend to be analytical and rational. In contrast, persons who are right-brain-dominant tend to be imaginative and artistic. Left-brained functioning is dominated by language and verbal reasoning, while right-brained functioning includes free-associative behavior and child-like creativity. Point out to the participants that, when listing possible solutions, they should first rely on right-brain functioning; that is, they should be as creative as possible without being critical. Often, as soon as a possible solution is proposed, there is a tendency to criticize and reject it before it can be expanded upon. Just as children have an unending capacity for using their imaginations without being critical, group members should consider all possible solutions before deciding whether they are practical.

Ask a volunteer to present his or her problem, stating it as specifically as possible and then writing it on the board. Then have that individual rate the problem on a scale from 0 to 10, with 0 signifying "not a problem" and 10 "a major problem that I worry about all the time." (Problems rated 10 are daily concerns that interfere with normal function.)

Have the group list possible solutions. They may discover that one solution triggers another idea. Remind the group that this is not the time to criticize the proposed solutions and that listing these ideas is a creative process. Allow enough time for the listing of as many solutions as possible. Then have the group discuss the positive or negative points for each solution and consider its positive and negative consequences. Remind participants to avoid pessimism and negative thinking, keeping an open mind.

Next ask the individual who presented the problem to choose the solutions that seem most helpful in solving it and to list these solutions under "Execute your solution" on the worksheet. Finally, have the volunteer save the worksheet so that he or she can rate the problem again after trying out the proposed solutions.

Some participants may find this technique contrived and artificial. Point out to them that, although it may not be the best technique for them, it conveys an important message: There are solutions to any problem, and each individual has the capacity to find at least partial solutions to what appear to be insurmountable problems. Encourage each participant to complete the worksheet for at least two problems.

WEIGHT MANAGEMENT AND NUTRITION

Weight management training is an integral part of any chronic pain program. Some patients have a strong desire to eat at the onset of pain; others completely lose their appetites. Pain patients are often reluctant to exercise because their pain increases in association with physical activity. Unfortunately, decreased activity is often accompanied by weight gain. The problem is exacerbated when a patient remains at home and passes time by eating.

Patients who are overweight and who have back pain may blame their obesity on their pain. Unfortunately, some health care professionals conversely blame the pain on the patient's obesity. In certain cases excessive weight gain may contribute to back problems. However, there is no consistent evidence in the literature to suggest that drastic weight loss alleviates chronic back pain.

Although maintaining a normal weight may not always lessen chronic pain, it can improve a person's self-image. Chronic pain tends to control every aspect of a patient's lifestyle, and excessive weight gain further undermines the patient's sense of control.

The group should discuss why chronic pain patients tend to gain weight and should consider the weight-gain formula in the patient's handbook (intake = output + storage). This equation can help group members appreciate the importance of proper diet and exercise.

There is indirect evidence that good nutrition helps to diminish pain. The group's discussion may focus on the benefit of vitamins, carbohydrates, and foods that influence certain pain conditions (e.g., fish oils sometimes decrease inflammation). Certain persons are at risk for dietary conditions that can aggravate a painful condition. Examples include alcoholics, persons over the age of 60 who have absorption problems, pregnant women, teenagers, and patients with cancer. Deficiencies in vitamins such as C, D, B1, and certain members of the B complex may contribute to painful symptoms.

A nutritionist should be invited to provide dietary information to the group and to inform patients about how best to improve the way they eat. Specific information on topics like low-fat foods and nutritional labels encourages careful food selection. Food diaries help pain patients to become aware of their eating habits. Patients should monitor their diets for up to 1 week and then consult with the nutritionist. Patients are typically asked to record all foods, fat grams, and calories eaten as well as information about the environmental, emotional, and behavioral contexts in which they eat. A sample daily food diary is presented on page 119.

Negative thoughts associated with diet and weight management often perpetuate poor eating habits. Self-statements that the patient believes are true may in fact reflect distorted ideas or irrational thoughts about control over eating behaviors. Examples of such statements include "When I start to eat, I have no control and can't stop" and "I am a failure for eating that dessert; I have no will power." Weight management is difficult for many individuals and the perception of failure is common. Patients should recognize that they can change their "negative self-talk" to make weight management easier. Group members should be asked to give examples of how they perpetuate negative perceptions of their eating behavior.

Patients who have a major weight problem and want advice about weight loss should consult with their physician and with a nutritionist. Valuable behavioral strategies are offered in the patient's handbook to help maintain weight. The handbook's general guidelines on eating and weight management should be discussed. Examples of high-fiber, low-fat foods should be offered (cereal, bagels, English muffins, brown rice, oatmeal, pasta, baked potatoes, raw and steamed vegetables, fruits, lean meats, fish, chicken, turkey, low-fat milk, yogurt, crackers, pretzels, licorice, jelly beans, and vanilla wafers). Textbooks on diet and nutrition should be consulted when necessary.

VOCATIONAL REHABILITATION

The goal of vocational rehabilitation is a return to work. After an extended period out of work, chronic pain patients become both physically and psychologically deconditioned to the demands and stresses of the workplace. In a pain management program, some time should be allotted to the discussion of back-to-work issues in a group setting. If possible, a vocational rehabilitation counselor should attend the group session and share information on resources with the members. Together, a vocational rehabilitation counselor and a patient can develop an individualized plan that incorporates both long-range employment goals and short-term objectives based on medical, psychological, social, and vocational factors. Vocational rehabilitation counselors are specialists in the assessment of aptitudes and interests, transferable skills, physical capacity, modifications in the workplace, skills training, and job readiness.

The number of recorded work-related disabilities has increased dramatically over the past 30 years. The return-to-work statistics are alarming. Chronic pain patients who have been out of work for longer than a year have an estimated chance of ever returning to full-time employment of < 3%; those who have been out of work for longer than 2 years have < 1% chance of ever working again. Insurance carriers are interested in the rehabilitation of these patients because of the enormous expenses the patients incur. An estimated 5% of all workers' compensation claimants account for 85% of the disability funds distributed. Unfortunately, many patients do not know what options they have for a return to work. It is helpful to review what a vocational rehabilitation counselor does and to help group members understand what is involved in a return-to-work determination.

Many chronic pain patients receive workers' compensation benefits or social security disability income. These patients may fear that their benefits will be jeopardized if they return to work. A vocational rehabilitation counselor can help a patient negotiate with an employer a return-to-work trial that will not jeopardize the patient's income. For example, the counselor can arrange with an employer to hire the patient for a specific period (e.g., 3 months) during which the employee's productivity will be evaluated. The employer agrees to pay the employee reduced wages that will not jeopardize workers' compensation. In addition, the employer agrees to train the individual and, at the conclusion of the work period, either to hire the individual full time or to write a letter of reference. In this way the patient gains work experience with a letter of reference without jeopardizing disability benefits. Advantages to the employer include the performance of work at lower wages with no obligation to hire on a permanent basis. The vocational rehabilitation counselor acts as a mediator in getting the chronic pain patient "in the door" of a business - and eventually, perhaps, back to work.

One common misconception is that persons receiving compensation benefits are lazy and are not interested in working. In fact, most people on disability leave wish that they were working. In our society work is a valuable part of who we are. We all have a need to accomplish things and to feel useful. Although many chronic pain patients may not have the option of returning to their former place of employment, they should be encouraged to explore other full-time, part-time, or volunteer work opportunities. Patients should become familiar with the Americans with Disabilities Act (ADA) so that they know their rights regarding discrimination due to a pain-related disability. The central theme of the ADA is that a disability that does not interfere with job performance cannot be used to reject applicants. In addition, employers are required to make accommodations for persons with disabilities so that they can work. An outline of the ADA is presented in the Appendix of the patient's handbook (pp. 215-216).

Local vocational resources should be discussed with the group. Patients may find it useful to have, for instance, information on the Job Training Partnership Act (with specific data on state and local funding), veterans' programs that help people return to work, and the vocational services offered by the Division of Industrial Accidents.

Patients may not be aware of one employment advantage of persons with disabilities. Some large corporations receive tax credits for disabled employees. Thus, individuals with chronic pain may want to consider contacting the disability/equal opportunity office of a corporation rather than the personnel department to improve their chances of being hired.

The facilitator or a vocational rehabilitation counselor should outline various aspects of the rehabilitation process at a group session. The components may include a vocational assessment, a transferable skills analysis, a physical capacity evaluation, a work disability assessment, a job analysis, and an employment readiness determination. The Vocational Issues Questionnaire on page 121 can be used to stimulate group discussion of return-to-work issues. The questionnaire covers issues such as pain persistence and belief in eventual return to work. Research shows that individuals are more likely to return to work if they believe that they will. The therapist should refer persons who believe that their chances of returning to full-time employment are > 50% for a vocational rehabilitation functional capacity test.

SPECIAL TOPICS

Pain is real when you get other people to believe in it. If no one believes in it but you, your pain is madness or hysteria.

Naomi Wolf

A number of special topics included in the patient's handbook may or may not be discussed in group sessions, depending on the length of the program and the importance of these issues to members of a particular group. They are not among the "core" issues in the program but are frequently of concern to chronic pain patients.

SEXUAL ISSUES

This topic is important to most patients who experience chronic pain but is rarely mentioned by other health professionals. Patients frequently report that they have had no sexual contact with their partner for months or even years because the act of making love increases their pain and the pain interferes with sexual enjoyment. They often express feelings of guilt about being unable to have a normal sexual relationship with their mate, and they consider themselves personally responsible for the lack of sexual contact. Although it must be acknowledged, this topic may be difficult to raise in a group setting since it is personal and private.

Group members should be told that sexual issues are a common concern among persons with persistent pain and should be asked how comfortable they feel about discussion of this topic. If some members prefer not to share their personal thoughts or experiences, it is still advisable to talk generally about how pain interferes with normal sexual functioning and to recommend open discussion with sexual partners. Patients should be told that they can participate in pleasurable sexual experiences with minimal pain if they share information, communicate openly with their partners, and experiment. The facilitator should list important issues surrounding pain and sexual dysfunction. Information presented in a matter-of-fact manner, interspersed with humor, is usually well received.

MEMORY AND CONCENTRATION

Patients with chronic pain frequently have problems with memory and concentration. Many question their sanity because they have difficulty remembering even the simplest things. Some suspect that they are developing Alzheimer's syndrome or wonder whether something is seriously wrong with their brains. Examples of short-term memory problems reported by patients include placing keys on a table and forgetting where they are minutes later, listening to a phone number or name and forgetting it seconds later, having to reread articles in newspapers and magazines, and forgetting whether medication has been taken.

Patients who enjoy reading are frustrated by their inability to concentrate when their pain is severe. This problem can be especially trying for patients in a retraining program who must sit for long periods and learn new information. Patients should be reassured that this is a common difficulty among persons with chronic pain. It should be pointed out that this situation is analogous to that in which someone tries to concentrate while a jackhammer is being used in the room next door. External "white noise" makes concentration and recall very difficult. Chronic pain patients have *internal* white noise that plays havoc with their concentration. Moreover, medications taken for pain can cloud cognitive processes and adversely affect memory. Anxiety related to pain also negatively influences concentration and memory.

Patients need to know that they are at risk for problems with concentration and memory because of their condition. These problems affect short-term more than long-term memory. Chronic pain patients must make an extra effort to remember information, using, for example, the memory "tricks" outlined in the patient's handbook.

HUMOR AND PAIN

Either this man is dead or my watch has stopped
Groucho Marx (taking the pulse of
someone who has just fainted at a
dinner party)

There is nothing more serious than pain and suffering. Words used to describe pain include torture, punishment, despair, penalty, torment, distress, misery, agony, and grief. All have a negative connotation. In some societies, chronic pain is thought to have some positive effects: It can strengthen a person and can make him or her more spiritual. In Western societies, however, chronic pain is considered to be an experience of no value that should be eliminated at all costs. When you are the one experiencing chronic pain, you may feel that there is no room for laughter.

However, some have argued that pain can and should be a laughing matter. In *Anatomy of an Illness as Perceived by the Patient*, Norman Cousins (1979) describes how he "laughed" his way out of a crippling disease. His theme is that everyone must take responsibility for his or her own recovery from a chronic illness and that mental attitude has a lot to do with that recovery. As Rene Dubos states in the book's introduction, "It is all but certain that active participation in the treatment, were it only through laughter or the cultivation of the will to live, as in Cousins' case, helps to mobilize the natural defense mechanisms of the patient which are the indispensable agents of recovery" (Cousins, 1979, pp. 22-23).

Humor can be used to manage pain in a number of ways. First, *humor is the antidote for feelings of hopelessness and despair*. The *American Heritage Dictionary* defines humor as the ability to perceive, enjoy, or express what is amusing, comical, incongruous, or absurd. Chronic pain patients tend to be strongly pessimistic and to have difficulty enjoying life or seeing hope for the future. They often carry feelings of anger, guilt, and resentment wherever they go. Humor is incompatible with these feelings and has a way of defusing negative thoughts and feelings.

Second, *humor increases one's sense of control*. Chronic pain undermines feelings of mastery and control; flare-ups are unpredictable and disability due to pain negatively impacts every aspect of life. Dr. Martin Seligman (1994), in his book *What You Can Change and What You Can't*, notes that cognitive therapy has little long-term effect on conditions such as sexual orientation, alcoholism, and dieting but can have a marked impact on depression, anger, and anxiety, and the misperceptions and thoughts that affect mood. Humor can be used in cognitive therapy as a coping technique and as a means of identifying irrational thoughts. It can help change the way a person thinks about failure and loss and promote a sense of control.

Third, *humor lends distance to any situation*. It is important to point out that laughing at yourself or others removes you from a situation long enough to gather a different perspective. There is a sense of being above the problem; when you are in pain, it helps to feel that you are outside of yourself, even for a moment. Humor can also distract you from pain and worried thoughts and help you become "objective" about troublesome situations.

Finally, *laughter has positive physiologic effects that help combat pain*. The research literature demonstrates that healing and immune function are improved in conjunction with feelings of well-being. Unexpressed anxiety, anger, and resentment can increase likelihood of heart disease, cancer, and poor immune function. Conversely, laughter can combat negative moods and exert a positive impact on health.

The use of humor to deal with pain entails some risks. For example, friends and family members may forget or disbelieve that a person who can laugh has "real" pain.

Each of the suggestions in Chapter 17 of the patient's handbook for improving mood and outlook on life should be reviewed with the group. Participants should be asked to share ways in which humor has been helpful for them and to suggest "one liners" that can be used in social situations. Laughter should be encouraged in the group itself. It may arise spontaneously or can be promoted by allotting time for humorous stories at the beginning of or the end of each session. It is important for the therapist to share humorous stories and to laugh with the group.

HOW TO BE "SMART" ABOUT PAIN

The adage that time heals all wounds may not apply for chronic pain patients. However, these individuals can learn ways to cope intelligently with pain over time. Being "smart" about pain means coming to terms with it instead of denying it or becoming totally defeated by it. Patients must learn to trust themselves to know the best thing to do; this self-trust comes with time and experience and can be taught like any skill.

The stages of change outlined by Dr. Elizabeth Kubler-Ross (1975) in her published work on death and dying are applicable to chronic pain as well. These stages are shock, denial, anger, depression, and acceptance. After experiencing the shock of a trauma, patients go to many health care professionals in the belief that someone will be able to get rid of their pain. They refuse to believe that they have a residual pain problem that cannot be resolved through modern medical technology. In other words, they are in denial. Most patients then go through periods of anger - either at themselves or at others - as they recognize that their condition is chronic and incurable. This anger is accompanied by periods of depression and hopelessness. Finally, patients come to terms with their situations. They neither continue to fight the problem, nor do they resign themselves in a helpless manner. They learn to know their limits and to accept them.

Pain patients usually go through stages of readiness to use pain management strategies. The therapist may recognize individuals in a group who are eager to understand and cope with their condition and no longer believe that a quick solution exists.

Chapter 18 of the patient's handbook offers common-sense tips on being smart about pain. This topic may invite considerable discussion. Group members should be encouraged to give concrete examples of how they have been "smart."

DEALING WITH THE MEDICAL SYSTEM

Patients must learn to be their own best advocates. To this end, they must become educated consumers who can get the best service from the medical system. They should be encouraged to speak up for themselves, gather information about possible treatments, and ask questions. They should participate in all decisions about their care. Since medical and rehabilitation centers have their own way of operating and since some centers may not welcome equal participation in treatment decisions, patients will benefit from a discussion of how to maximize their input into the medical system. This discussion should cover the training and background of persons in the various health care disciplines involved in treating chronic pain. It is useful to identify biases among health care professionals on controversial topics such as chronic opioid therapy, workers' compensation, repeat testing, second opinions, and the relative value of invasive procedures versus behavioral techniques.

The points outlined in this section in the patient's handbook can help avert problems between the health care provider and the person with chronic pain. There is a risk that a discussion of this topic will generate complaints about how medical professionals have mismanaged care or how health care providers have not understood pain. Some expression of discontent can be helpful, but continual complaining should be discouraged. Group members should be encouraged to offer one another advice and input on possible solutions to problems related to getting help from the medical system.

SOCIAL SUPPORT

Perceived support is an important mediating factor in coping with pain. Many of the patients referred to a pain program have limited outside support. There is evidence that individuals with poor perceived support (e.g., those who make statements such as "No one understands what I am going through" or "My family members often ignore or become angry with me") have the most difficulty in coping with pain. Often these patients report feelings of isolation and abandonment.

Group members should complete the Social Support Questionnaire at the end of Chapter 20 in the patient's handbook and score their responses. Open discussion of social support issues is important. Participants should have an opportunity to share the ways in which they deal with feelings of isolation. Each member should discuss approaches he or she has tried in order to increase social-support networks at home and in the community. A plan of action should be devised for use after completion of the program. Group members who have few family members or friends may have trouble coming up with a plan.

Certain patients may need to discuss issues centered around their pain and their religious or spiritual beliefs. This type of discussion is healthy and should be encouraged. If the facilitator does not feel comfortable addressing spiritual questions raised by group members, he or she should be prepared to refer these individuals to someone who can do so. Many persons with chronic pain can gain a sense of peace and positive acceptance of their condition with pastoral counseling. Prayer and religious counseling have been shown to decrease anxiety and contribute to a general sense of purpose and well-being.

   Patients should also be encouraged to contact outside organizations to learn more about managing their pain and to maintain contact with others. Unfortunately, patients in leaderless support groups sometimes receive misinformation or become overly zealous in the cause of informing the general public about their specific pain problem. It is helpful for the facilitator to maintain ties with all group members after completion of the structured pain program in order to offer guidance about which organizations and support groups are best. Table 5.2 (below) provides a list of national associations that members may contact for additional information about pain support groups and relevant publications on pain in the United States.

TABLE 5.2: ASSOCIATIONS WITH INFORMATION ABOUT PAIN SUPPORT GROUPS AND RELEVANT PUBLICATIONS ON PAIN IN THE UNITED STATES

---

1. *Agency for Healthcare Policy and Research Publications Clearinghouse*
    PO Box 8547
    Silver Spring, MD 20907
    (800) 358-9295

2. *American Academy of Pain Medicine*
    4700 W. Lake Avenue
    Glenview, IL 60025-1485
    (847) 375-4731

3. *American Pain Society*
    4700 W. Lake Avenue
    Glenview, IL 60025-1485
    (847) 375-4715

4. *American Council for Headache Education*
    875 Kings Highway, Suite 200
    West Deptford, NJ 08096
    (800) 255-ACHE

5. *American Chronic Pain Association*
    PO Box 850
    Rocklin, CA 95677
    (916) 632-0922

6. *Arthritis Foundation*
    1314 Spring Street
    Atlanta, GA 30309
    (404) 872-7100

7. *Committee on Pain Therapy*
    American Society of Anesthesiologists
    515 Busse Highway
    Park Ridge, IL 60068
    (708) 825-5586

Table 5.2 *(Continued)*

8. ***Commission on Accreditation of Rehabilitation Facilities***
   2500 N. Pantano Road, Suite 226
   Tucson, AZ 85715
   (602) 748-1212

9. ***Fibromyalgia Network***
   5700 Stockdale Highway, Suite 100
   Bakersfield, CA 93309
   (805) 631-1950

10. ***International Association for the Study of Pain***
    909 NE 43rd Street, Room 306
    Seattle, WA 98105-6020
    (206) 547-6409

11. ***National Chronic Pain Outreach Association***
    7979 Old Georgetown Road, Suite 100
    Bethesda, MD 20814
    (301) 652-4948

12. ***National Headache Foundation***
    5252 North Western Avenue
    Chicago, IL 60625
    (800) 523-8858 - in Illinois
    (800) 843-2256 - other states

13. ***National Cancer Institute***
    Office of Cancer Communications
    Building 31, Room 10-24
    Bethesda, MD 20892
    (800) 4-CANCER

14. ***Pain Management Information Center***
    401 Harris B Dates Drive
    Ithaca, NY 14850
    (800) 322-7642

15. ***Wisconsin Cancer Pain Initiative***
    1300 University Avenue, Room 3675
    Madison, WI 53706
    (608) 262-0978

RELAPSE PREVENTION

The topic of relapse prevention should be discussed during one of the last sessions of the structured program. Some patients believe that completion of a pain management program will protect them from future problems and that their condition will continue to improve. They believe that they will no longer have to face setbacks or flare-ups. It is important to point out that everyone in the group will probably experience a *lapse* in his or her condition - that is, a short-term setback that may include increased pain and decreased activity.   However, the hope is that no one will have a *relapse* (i.e., a return of problematic symptoms and negative behaviors that perpetuate the pain syndrome, such as increased pain, prolonged inactivity, depression, over-reliance on medication, and negative self-statements).   A lapse is a temporary state that can lead to a relapse.   The group's facilitator can illustrate these concepts by drawing a graph that shows a positive linear trend upward with peaks and valleys.   The low points represent lapses.   A reversal of the trend, with the return of the line to the bottom of the chart, would represent a relapse (see Figure 5.2 below).

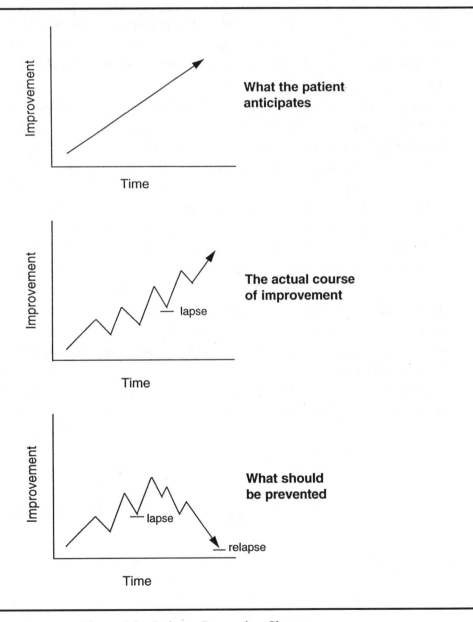

Figure 5.2.   Relapse Prevention Charts.

The two scenarios in Chapter 21 (pp. 187-188) in the patient's handbook should be read and discussed. Group members should be asked to define what a lapse and a relapse mean for them, to complete the relapse-prevention worksheet (p. 191), and to discuss how they can tell if they are experiencing a lapse and what they can do to get out of it. Participants should share their ideas about relapse prevention and should create an individual relapse-prevention plan to use when they have a setback.

An estimated 30% to 70% of patients with chronic pain experience a relapse of their condition within 1 year after completing a pain management program. This information is both encouraging and discouraging; many people benefit from the program but continue to need treatment for their pain. Factors that are believed to influence relapse include patients' beliefs about their condition, their home and work environments, their use (or lack of use) of pain management strategies, economic and compensation issues, and content of the pain management program.

Many techniques for preventing a relapse have been reported in the behavior literature. These include setting specific short- and long-range goals; identifying situations that place the patient at risk for a flare-up; coming up with a relapse-prevention plan; reviewing pain-management strategies; encouraging participation in booster sessions and follow-up support groups; including family members in treatment and follow-up; combining medical, psychological, and vocational therapies in a multidisciplinary setting; and offering professional support when needed. Relapse of a chronic-pain condition is a multifactorial problem that can be only partially controlled. All strategies that will maximize continued benefit from participation in a structured group program should be considered.

Discussion of relapse prevention should be coupled with an overview of the pain management strategies listed in Chapter 22 of the patient's handbook. In order to maintain the gains made in the program, patients will need to incorporate these strategies into their daily routine. Group members can share the methods - both those from the patient's handbook and their own ideas - that work best for them. It is important to point out that pain management requires changes in lifestyle. Patients tend to revert to negative pain behaviors and must plan ways to prevent themselves from doing so.

SAMPLE EXERCISE RECORD

Directions: This form should be used to monitor your exercise. Please circle whether you stretched before and after each exercise session. Include the date and type of exercise and check the combined time you spent exercising.

Name: *Joe Schmoe*   Start Date: *4/1*   Record #: *1*

Day	1	2	3	4	5	6	7	8	9	10
Warm-Up Stretching	(Y)	(Y)	(Y)	(Y)	Y	Y	Y	(Y)	Y	Y
Cool-Down Stretching	Y	Y	(Y)	(Y)	(Y)	(Y)	(Y)	(Y)	(Y)	(Y)

Minutes of Cardiovascular Activity

Date:	4/1	4/2	4/3	4/4	4/5	4/6	4/7	4/8	4/9	4/10
Activity:	walking	walking/exercise bike	walking	swimming	walking/bike	walking	walking/swimming	walking	bike/treadmill	speed walking

EXERCISE RECORD

Directions: This form should be used to monitor your exercise. Please circle whether you stretched before and after each exercise session. Include the date and type of exercise and check the combined time you spent exercising.

Name: _____ Start Date: _____ Record #: _____

Day	1	2	3	4	5	6	7	8	9	10
Warm-Up Stretching	Y	Y	Y	Y	Y	Y	Y	Y	Y	Y
Cool-Down Stretching	Y	Y	Y	Y	Y	Y	Y	Y	Y	Y

Minutes of Cardiovascular Activity

```
20  .    .    .    .    .    .    .    .    .    .

15  .    .    .    .    .    .    .    .    .    .

10  .    .    .    .    .    .    .    .    .    .

 5  .    .    .    .    .    .    .    .    .    .

 0  .    .    .    .    .    .    .    .    .    .
```

Date: ___ ___ ___ ___ ___ ___ ___ ___ ___ ___

Activity:

PAIN MANAGEMENT CENTER
SAMPLE OPIOID THERAPY CONTRACT
<u>INFORMED CONSENT FORM</u>

The following agreement relates to my use of controlled substances for chronic pain prescribed by a physician at the Pain Management Center at Brigham and Women's Hospital. I recognize that specific policies regarding the use of controlled substances are followed by the staff at the Pain Management Center. I will be provided with controlled substances while actively participating in this program only if I adhere to the following regulations:

1. I will use the substances only within the parameters given by the Pain Management Center physician.
2. I will not receive replacements for lost or stolen medications.
3. I will receive controlled substances only from the Brigham and Women's pain staff. My violation of this will result in a discontinuation of treatment.
4. I will not expect to receive additional medication before my next scheduled refill, even if my prescription runs out.
5. I will accept generic brands of my prescription medication.
6. If it appears to the physician that my daily functioning and quality of life are not benefiting from treatment with the controlled substance, I will gradually taper my medication as prescribed by the physician. I will not hold any member of the Pain Management Center liable for problems caused by discontinuance of controlled substances, provided that I receive 30 days notice of termination.
7. I agree to submit to urine and blood screening to detect the use of nonprescribed medications at any time.
8. I recognize that my chronic pain represents a complex problem that may benefit from physical therapy, psychotherapy, and behavioral medicine strategies. I also recognize that my participation in the management of my pain is extremely important. I agree to actively participate in all aspects of the Pain Management Program to maximize the likelihood that my level of functioning will increase and my ability to cope with my condition will improve.

_Anna Felaxis_____   _6/24/96_____
Patient Signature   Date

_Seymour Butz, M.D._____   _6-24-96_____
Physician Signature   Date

_José Felaxis_____   _6/25/96_____
Family Member or Significant Other Signature   Date

SAMPLE MEDICATION RECORD

Name: _Fred Jones_   Date: _10/24_

Directions: Please fill out this sheet for the next 7 days. List all the drugs you take each day, the milligrams (mg), and the number of pills or capsules you take per day. List any "over-the-counter" drugs you take, such as aspirin, Bufferin, Tylenol, and so forth.

Date	Name of Drug	Number of Milligrams (mg)	Number of Pills or Capsules Taken Each Day
Monday 10/24	Elavil	100 mg	1
	Motrin	800 mg	3
Tuesday 10/25	Elavil	100 mg	1
	Motrin	800 mg	3
	Percocet		2
Wednesday 10/26	Elavil	100 mg	1
	Motrin	800 mg	3
Thursday 10/27	Elavil	100 mg	1
	Motrin	800 mg	3
	Benadryl	50 mg	3
Friday 10/28	Elavil	100 mg	1
	Motrin	800 mg	3
	Tylenol	500 mg	2
Saturday 10/29	Elavil	100 mg	1
	Motrin	800 mg	3
Sunday 10/30	Elavil	100 mg	1
	Motrin	800 mg	3
	Tylenol	500 mg	2

MEDICATION RECORD

Name: _____   Date:_____

Directions: Please fill out this sheet for the next 7 days. List all the drugs you take each day, the milligrams (mg), and the number of pills or capsules you take per day. List any "over-the-counter" drugs you take, such as aspirin, Bufferin, Tylenol, and so forth.

Date	Name of Drug	Number of Milli-grams (mg)	Number of Pills or Capsules Taken Each Day
Monday			
Tuesday			
Wednesday			
Thursday			
Friday			
Saturday			
Sunday			

SIDE EFFECTS CHECKLIST

Name: _____   Date: _____

Directions: Please identify any adverse effects you have experienced within the past 24 hours by rating the following symptoms from 0 = absent to 3 = severe.

Symptom	Absent	Mild	Moderate	Severe
1. Drowsiness	0	1	2	3
2. Dizziness	0	1	2	3
3. Anxiety	0	1	2	3
4. Muddled Thinking	0	1	2	3
5. Coordination Impairment	0	1	2	3
6. Irritability/Weird Feeling	0	1	2	3
7. Depression	0	1	2	3
8. Weakness/Sluggishness	0	1	2	3
9. Headache	0	1	2	3
10. Memory Lapse	0	1	2	3
11. Dry Mouth	0	1	2	3
12. Visual Distortions	0	1	2	3
13. Nausea/Vomiting	0	1	2	3
14. Sweating	0	1	2	3
15. Constipation	0	1	2	3
16. Heart Palpitations	0	1	2	3
17. Itching	0	1	2	3
18. Breathing Problems	0	1	2	3
19. Nightmares	0	1	2	3
20. Difficulty Urinating	0	1	2	3

SAMPLE SLEEP DIARY

Directions: Please monitor your sleep behavior each day for 1 week. Complete each section in this diary.

DAYS	1	2	3	4	5	6	7
DATE	10/20	10/21	10/22	10/23	10/24	10/25	10/26
Avoided Day Naps (Y/N)	Y	N	N	N	Y	Y	Y
Exercised (Y/N)	Y	Y	Y	Y	Y	Y	Y
Avoided Stimulants (Y/N)	Y	Y	N	N	Y	Y	Y
Avoided Sleeping Medication (Y/N)	Y	N	N	N	Y	Y	Y
Relaxed Before Bed (Y/N)	Y	N	Y	Y	Y	Y	Y
Used Distraction Techniques (Y/N)	Y	Y	N	N	Y	Y	Y
Kept to a Schedule (Y/N)	Y	N	N	N	Y	Y	Y
Time to Bed (e.g., 11:00 p.m.)	10:00 p.m.	10:00 p.m.	10:30 p.m.	11:30 p.m.	10:00 p.m.	10:00 p.m.	10:00 p.m.
Minutes to Get to Sleep	30	45	2 hrs.	1 hr.	45	30	30
Times Awake During the Night (0-4)	3	2	2	3	2	1	1
Total Sleeping Time (Hours)	3	3	4	5½	7	6	6
SLEEP SCORE (use scale below):	1	0	1	2	3	3-4	3

(0 = Very Poor; 1 = Poor; 2 = Fair; 3 = Good; 4 = Excellent)

SLEEP DIARY

Directions: Please monitor your sleep behavior each day for 1 week. Complete each section in this diary.

(Example)

DAYS	1	1	2	3	4	5	6	7
DATE	10/20							
Avoided Day Naps (Y/N)	Y							
Exercised (Y/N)	Y							
Avoided Stimulants (Y/N)	Y							
Avoided Sleeping Medication (Y/N)	N							
Relaxed Before Bed (Y/N)	Y							
Used Distraction Techniques (Y/N)	Y							
Kept to a Schedule (Y/N)	Y							
Time to Bed (e.g., 11:00 p.m.)	10:00 p.m.							
Minutes to Get to Sleep	30							
Times Awake During the Night (0-4)	3							
Total Sleeping Time (Hours)	4 ½							
SLEEP SCORE (use scale below):	2							

(0 = Very Poor; 1 = Poor; 2 = Fair; 3 = Good; 4 = Excellent)

SAMPLE SOLVE-PROBLEMS WORKSHEET*

Name: _Joe Schmoe_   Date: _11/20_

Problem Rating Scale:

0 . . . 1 . . . 2 . . . 3 . . . 4 . . . 5 . . . 6 . . . 7 . . . 8 . . . 9 . . . 10
Not at all a problem   Very much a problem

Problem Rating: ___8___

1. **S**tate the problem:

I have difficulty doing any lifting at work.

2. **O**utline the problem: Part of my job is to move some boxes of paper from our office to the office across the hall. By the end of the day my pain is at its worst, but I don't like letting others know I am in pain.

3. **L**ist possible solutions:	4. **V**iew the consequences:
a. I could ask my friend Joe to lift the boxes on the days when my back hurts the most.	a. + Joe is always willing to help. - I don't want to rely on others.
b. I could ask my boss to change my job so I won't have to lift the boxes.	b. + This would solve the problem. - I don't want my boss to know about my back pain; others may resent me.

c. I could move the boxes in the morning when I am better able to do it.	c. + I would be in better condition to lift. - Sometimes the boxes are needed in the afternoon.
d. I could get a trolly or dolly to use when moving the boxes.	d. + This would save me from a lot of pain. - A trolly would be awkward and I would need a place to store it.
e. I could rest during my lunch break so my back wouldn't hurt so much.	e. + I would be rested for the afternoon. - Sometimes I don't get a chance to rest.
f. I could meet with a physical therapist to learn proper ways to lift and exercises to build up my back muscles.	f. + The instruction and exercise would be helpful. - It would take time and money to see the PT regularly.

5. Execute your solution: Executed solutions a, c, d, and f. Joe has agreed to help me and the physical therapist has been very helpful.

Problem Rating After Executing the Solutions: _3_

SOLVE-PROBLEMS WORKSHEET

Name: _____   Date:_____

Problem Rating Scale:

0 . . . 1 . . . 2 . . . 3 . . . 4 . . . 5 . . . 6 . . . 7 . . . 8 . . . 9 . . . 10
Not at all a problem   Very much a problem

Problem Rating: _____

1. State the problem:

2. Outline the problem:

3. List possible solutions: a.	4. View the consequences: a. +
	-
b.	b. +
	-

c. | c. +

                                        -

d. | d. +

                                        -

e. | e. +

                                        -

f. | f. +

                                        -

5.   **E**xecute your solution:

_____

Problem Rating After Executing the Solutions: _____

SAMPLE DAILY FOOD DIARY

Name: _____Fred Figure_____   Date: ___10/28___

Directions: Please record everything that you eat throughout the day. Enter the time that you eat it, your level of hunger, a brief description of the food and amount, whether you ate it as part of a meal, and your level of pain.

	Time	Hunger* 1-5	Food Description	Amount	Meal (Y/N)	Pain 0-10
1.	9:00 A.M.	2	English Muffin w/ Jelly	1	Y	3
2.	9:00 A.M.	2	Coffee and Orange Juice	1 cup each	Y	3
3.	12:00 P.M.	4	Hamburger w/ Lettuce + Tomato	Large	Y	5
4.	12:00 P.M.	4	French Fries	Regular	Y	5
5.	12:00 P.M.	4	Diet Coke	12 oz.	Y	5
6.	3:30 P.M.	3	Oatmeal Cookies	2	N	6
7.	3:30 P.M.	3	Diet Coke	12 oz.	N	6
8.	6:00 P.M.	4	Baked Chicken	3 oz.	Y	6
9.	6:00 P.M.	4	Noodles	½ cup	Y	6
10.	6:00 P.M.	4	Green Beans	½ cup	Y	6
11.	6:00 P.M.	4	Vanilla Frozen Yogurt	½ cup	Y	6
12.	9:30 P.M.	2	Popcorn w/ margarine	2 cups/1oz.	N	4
13.	9:30 P.M.	2	Diet Ginger Ale	6 oz.	N	4
14.	11:00 P.M.	2	2% Milk	6 oz.	N	4
15.						

*1 = Not Hungry; 5 = Extremely Hungry

DAILY FOOD DIARY

Name: _____   Date:_____

Directions: Please record everything that you eat throughout the day. Enter the time that you eat it, your level of hunger, a brief description of the food and amount, whether you ate it as part of a meal, and your level of pain.

	Time	Hunger* 1-5	Food Description	Amount	Meal (Y/N)	Pain 0-10
1.						
2.						
3.						
4.						
5.						
6.						
7.						
8.						
9.						
10.						
11.						
12.						
13.						
14.						
15.						

*1 = Not Hungry; 5 = Extremely Hungry

VOCATIONAL ISSUES QUESTIONNAIRE

1. How certain am I that my pain will persist for the next 5 years?

0	1	2	3	4	5	6	7	8	9	10
Very Uncertain					Moderately Certain					Very Certain

2. How certain am I that I will be employed within the next 5 years?

0	1	2	3	4	5	6	7	8	9	10
Very Uncertain					Moderately Certain					Very Certain

3. How certain am I that I can now do what was required of me in my former job?

0	1	2	3	4	5	6	7	8	9	10
Very Uncertain					Moderately Certain					Very Certain

4. How certain am I that I can learn new skills and adjust to my pain to get a "good" job?

0	1	2	3	4	5	6	7	8	9	10
Very Uncertain					Moderately Certain					Very Certain

5. Realistically, my chances of ever getting a full-time job are (0% to 100%) _____%.

6. The main factors that keep me from seeking and getting a full-time job are

    a.

    b.

    c.

    d.

    e.

CHAPTER 6

Program Evaluation

Accountability and "quality control" of pain centers in the future depend on developing a standardized assessment of treatment program effectiveness that is objective, quantifiable and reproducible.

S. Vasudevan, 1988

WHAT IS PROGRAM EVALUATION?

There has been a rapid change in the way health care services are offered in the United States. More and more decisions about treatment are made by employees of insurance carriers on the basis of financial resources rather than need. "Managed care" favors structured, group-based programs because they are time-limited and economical to run. However, the increasing need for accountability and efficacy has encouraged the implementation of cost-saving measures and ongoing evaluation. Preference is given to programs that are of demonstrated efficacy and are tailored to the individual (e.g., not all participants receive every treatment).

Program evaluation improves the use of resources, organizes data for marketing, and helps managers decide which direction a program will take. Effective program evaluation reports offer data to assist top level administrators to create solutions for poor outcome, increased costs, and decreased market share. The goals of program evaluation in chronic pain management programs are to increase the benefits to persons the program serves, increase program productivity, and improve market position.

An important component of any group-based pain program is its ability to measure its own effectiveness. A number of recommendations for effective program evaluation have been put forward by the Commission on Accreditation of Rehabilitation Facilities (CARF; 1994). Each program should have a mission statement and lists detailing admission criteria, services offered, specific objectives, the priority of each objective, expectations regarding minimal and optimal goals, objective measures of performance, the period to which these measures apply, and the way in which information collected is documented.

A system should be in place for obtaining follow-up information from patients on the use of medications, the use of health care services, return to gainful employment, functional activities, the ability to manage pain, and the subjective intensity of pain. This system should include a schedule for periodic contact with the patient after discharge and a data base containing information updated on a regular basis. This type of system helps determine how a program meets the needs of individual patients and of participants overall.

Program evaluation should encompass goals and objectives that are achievable and end results that are measurable. Each program evaluation system should include objectives and measures for (a) productivity of patients (e.g., return to work), (b) health care utilization (e.g., reduction in physician visits), (c) activity level (e.g., increased walking and exercising), (d) medication usage (e.g., adherence to AMA guidelines for proper use of medications), (e) program costs (e.g., maintenance of estimated and actual costs per patient at a steady level), (f) program productivity (e.g., a low ratio between the number of staff hours devoted to the program and the number of patient hours), (g) patient helpfulness ratings (e.g., above-average ratings of helpfulness for all services rendered), (h) pain coping and emotional adjustment (e.g., decreased ratings on the Beck Depression Inventory before and after treatment), (i) medical findings (e.g., improvement in objective physical measures, such as range of motion), and (j) socialization and activities of daily living (e.g., improved scores on the Sickness Impact Profile). A program evaluation report should include primary objectives, measures, time of measurement, source of information, and expectations as well as outcomes. Finally, program evaluation should help identify which services are most effective in the treatment of chronic pain patients.

Additional components of a program evaluation system include (a) follow-up data from a representative sample of patients, (b) valid and reliable dependent measures standardized for persons with pain, (c) a comparison of posttreatment and follow-up data, and (d) assessment of individual differences. An example of a program evaluation report based on data collected at the Pain Management Center at Brigham and Women's Hospital in Boston is provided on pages 129-133. The Helpfulness Questionnaire, used to collect treatment helpfulness data, was created by Stanley Chapman, PhD (Chapman, Jamison, & Sanders [unpublished]), and is presented on pages 135-137.

WHEN PROGRAMS DON'T WORK

Part of the reason that pain programs are perceived not to work is that everyone has a different definition of success. The patient wants the pain to stop. The referring physician wants a resolution of the patient's treatment. Family members want the patient to be the way he or she was before the pain problem developed. The patient's employer wants someone who is completely healthy with no threat of reinjury. Insurance claim representatives, when involved, want a quick settlement of the case. Unfortunately, problems often persist despite marked improvement in a patient's pain and sense of well-being. The expectation that a short pain program will reverse this process is unrealistic.

The following are reasons some pain programs have lower success rates than others: (a) all patients are accepted, (b) there are no clear goals or end points, (c) there are no expectations for participation, (d) patients are not given feedback about their performance, and (d) there is no formal follow-up. Some patients tend to regress to their initial behaviors after completing a behaviorally based pain program. Although this tendency may be inevitable, it is important to maintain follow-up contact and to hold support group sessions or "reunions" for persons who have completed an outpatient, group-based pain program in order to make relapse less likely. Patients who have completed a pain program should be given a specific schedule of return visits at which they can assess their progress.

MARKETING ISSUES

Pain management programs are small businesses and should operate as such. As with any small business, it is important to have a marketing plan. Whether a stand-alone proprietary organization or a part of a larger medical complex, each pain center should have a marketing strategy for the recruitment of both providers and patients. Elements in the development of a marketing plan include an analysis of current services, with the identification of strengths and weaknesses; an assessment of local competition; and the creation of a list of short- and long-term objectives.

ANALYSIS OF SERVICES

Members of the pain center should draft a mission statement. This process helps clarify the direction of the program and identify the persons being served. Information included in a program evaluation report is relevant to this effort. It is important to demonstrate that the services offered are effective. Attempts should be made to identify those carriers and providers who use your services and to list the referring physicians. Marketing studies suggest that efforts to increase the level of satisfaction among current referral sources have a greater impact on the number of referrals than efforts to market the program to the general public. The development of helpfulness questionnaires (see pp. 135-137) designed specifically for referring physicians or insurance carriers is recommended.

Before promoting the center's services to others it is important to identify its strengths and weaknesses. It is important to know what patients value and what they dislike about the center. Patients' degree of satisfaction with regard to the reception and support staff, waiting time, comfort and cleanliness of the facility, location and transportation issues, and clinic hours should be solicited and analyzed.

ASSESSMENT OF THE COMPETITION

A list of comparable local services that meet the needs of patients with chronic pain should be compiled. The strengths and weaknesses of each facility on this list should be identified. A greater awareness of the local competition helps to define the local market share for pain management services.

DELINEATION OF OBJECTIVES

A marketing strategy should have both short- and long-term goals. These may include an increase in the number of referrals, a decrease in overall program expenses, an increase in services requested by patients and providers, an improvement in patient satisfaction, and an increase in reimbursements.

DEVELOPMENT OF A STRATEGY

After marketing objectives have been listed a marketing strategy needs to be created. It may be important for the administrator of a pain management program to attend marketing courses and seminars in order to gain a better understanding of the business workings of a pain management center. The vehicles used in marketing include advertising (e.g., through newspapers and the yellow pages), organizing public lectures or talks, mailing brochures and referral information, creating a monthly newsletter, and publishing the results of studies of patients attending the pain management center. Each marketing plan should have a budget to cover the expenses incurred.

There are a number of interesting statistics which impact marketing practices of health care services: (a) The average business never hears from 96% of its unhappy customers, (b) the average customer who has a problem tells 9 to 10 people, (c) customers whose complaints are resolved tell 5 people, (d) most referrals are generated because someone trusts someone else, (e) most referrals are generated from persons with whom one has regular contact, and (f) 25% of referring sources account for 75% of referrals.

Marketing is an ongoing process in which objectives are redefined and programmatic changes are made. Newspaper, television, media coverage, yellow page listings, and direct mailings are important marketing strategies.

There are a number of suggestions to consider when looking to improve a clinical practice: (a) Join a group practice with a shared central administration, (b) invest in practice management software, (c) invest in modes of electronic communication and explore medical communication packages which offer capability for electronic claims, (d) have customized release and informed consent statements, (e) make business decisions recognizing that decisions made by consensus are not always the best, (f) promote the services to managed care companies and to individual employers, (g) call every referral source to get feedback about the services and learn ways to improve their value, (h) create a marketing plan for today and one for 2 years from now, and (i) be creative about each of the treatments.

In summary, marketing is the process of broadcasting to patients and service professionals the noteworthy aspects of your program. Although program qualities should be presented in the best light, the information provided must be absolutely accurate, and the extent of services offered should not be exaggerated.

SAMPLE PROGRAM EVALUATION REPORT
Pain Management Program
Brigham and Women's Hospital

GOALS OF THE PROGRAM

The Pain Management Program at Brigham and Women's Hospital is a 10-week multidisciplinary outpatient program for persons with chronic pain. This program is a component of the Pain Management Center under the Department of Anesthesia. It is designed to rehabilitate chronic pain patients, with the goals of reducing pain intensity, increasing physical functioning, promoting return to a productive lifestyle, and limiting future health care utilization. The program is time limited and includes patient education, progressive physical exercise, medication management, individual and group psychotherapy, family sessions, and relaxation training. The structured program is dedicated to providing rehabilitation services to persons with chronic pain so that they may live more satisfying lives.

ADMISSION CRITERIA

- Patient is referred by a physician or other medical professional.
- Patient can be treated on an outpatient basis.
- No evidence exists of a severe, untreated psychiatric condition.
- Patient has reached stabilized medical condition.
- Pain interferes with lifestyle functioning and contributes to emotional distress.
- Patient is physically and mentally able to attend and participate in an outpatient program.
- Reimbursement criteria have been identified.
- Patient is willing to learn pain management strategies.

SERVICES OFFERED

- Medical assessment
- Psychological assessment
- Relaxation training
- Patient education groups
- Individual and group psychotherapy
- Nerve blocks

- Biofeedback therapy
- Individual and group exercise
- Family conference sessions
- Drug prescriptions
- Follow-up group sessions

PATIENT DEMOGRAPHIC DATA

A sample of 60 pain patients who completed the structured outpatient pain management program at Brigham and Women's Hospital between January 1993 and January 1994 was included in this study. Ages ranged between 19 and 61 years (mean, 39.8; standard deviation, 9.9); 51.7% were males, 84.7% had completed high school, 46.7% were married, and 10.0% were employed either part-time or full-time. Eighty percent of participants were receiving workers' compensation. The average duration of pain was 46.8 months (standard deviation, 49.5) Seventy-three percent of patients stated that their pain was constant. The average pretreatment pain ratings on a 0 to 10 scale was 7.1.

PRIMARY PAIN SITE

The following primary pain sites were represented: low back, 43.3%; upper extremity, 16.7%; lower extremity, 15.0%; cervical back, 14.4%; head, 4.6%; pelvis/groin, 3.9%; myofascial (no primary site), 2.1%.

PATIENT HELPFULNESS RATINGS

Sixty patients completed the Posttreatment Helpfulness Questionnaire* on the day of discharge. Forty-six patients (77%) completed the Follow-Up Helpfulness Questionnaire 3 to 6 months after discharge. All treatments were rated on a visual analog scale. Each treatment was scored based on the following scale: -5 = Extremely harmful; 0 = Neutral; +5 = Extremely helpful.

TREATMENT HELPFULNESS DATA		
Treatment Description	Posttreatment Ratings $N = 60$	3- to 6-Month Follow-Up Ratings $N = 46$
Whole program	3.6	3.3
Group therapy sessions	3.4	3.2
Psychological assessment and treatment	3.1	3.3
Individual psychotherapy	3.1	3.1
Education group sessions	2.9	2.9
Relaxation training	2.7	2.2
Group exercise	2.5	1.8
Physical therapy assessment and treatment	2.4	1.6
Family group sessions	2.3	2.4
Drug prescriptions	2.1	2.6
Biofeedback	2.0	2.5
Medical assessment and treatment	1.7	2.6
Nerve blocks	1.2	0.7

GOALS AND OBJECTIVES

Pretreatment goals and objectives were established according to the Commission on Accreditation of Rehabilitation Facilities criteria. Minimum and maximum outcome expectancies were determined for

*Note. From *The Treatment Helpfulness Questionnaire: A Measure of Patient Satisfaction With Treatment Modalities Provided in Chronic Pain Management Programs*, by S. L. Chapman, R. N. Jamison, and S. H. Sanders, unpublished manuscript. (See example on pp. 135-137.)

each goal and were weighted for relative importance. Outcome results were based on Helpfulness Questionnaire data.

Goals	Objectives	Expectancies Min - Max	Relative Importance	Outcome
1. Decrease pain ratings	% of patients reporting lower pain ratings of 20% or more	Min 30% Max 60%	10%	39% of patients reported a decrease in pain 3 to 6 months after treatment
2. Increase up-time	% of patients reporting increased standing and sitting by 20% or more	Min 60% Max 90%	25%	73% of patients reported increased up-time
3. Improve coping	% of patients reporting improved coping on the coping items	Min 50% Max 80%	15%	43% of patients reported good to excellent coping 3 to 6 months after discharge
4. Improve sleep	% of patients reporting improved sleep on the sleeping item	Min 60% Max 80%	10%	63% of patients reported improved sleep 3 to 6 months after discharge
5. Improve return-to-work percentage	% of patients reporting return to paid work or in retraining program	Min 30% Max 50%	15%	24% of patients who planned to return to work did so 3 to 6 months after discharge
6. Decrease health care utilization	% of patients reporting hospitalizations or surgeries after discharge	Min 5% Max 15%	15%	7% of patients reported being hospitalized for their pain after discharge
7. Contain standard program costs	% of patients exceeding estimated costs of program	Min 5% Max 25%	10%	6% of patients exceeded estimated costs for treatment

FOLLOW-UP PAIN RATINGS

Pretreatment pain ratings on a scale of 0 to 10 averaged 7.1 (standard deviation, 1.6). Three to 6 months after discharge, mean pain ratings averaged 6.2 (standard deviation, 1.3).

ACTIVITY LEVEL

Overall 72.9% of patients stated that their level of activity had increased since they had completed the pain management program. The average number of hours per day standing or walking was 3.5 before treatment and 5.2 thereafter.

ABILITY TO COPE

Before the program, 12.2% of patients stated that their ability to cope with their pain was either good or excellent. By the end of the program 43.2% agreed with this statement.

SLEEP DISTURBANCES

On follow-up, 62.5% of respondents reported that their sleep was either slightly or significantly better.

RETURN TO WORK

Before the program, 15.3% of the patients were working either part-time or full-time. On follow-up, 23.8% of the patients stated that they were either working or actively involved in a retraining program.

HEALTH CARE UTILIZATION

On follow-up, 7.1% of patients stated that they had been hospitalized because of their pain, 2.4% stated that they had surgery for their pain, and 45.7% stated that they had not seen any health care professionals for their pain since discharge from the pain program.

FOLLOW-UP PLANS

Of those polled, 77.1% stated that plans for follow-up were adequate.

AVERAGE COST OF PROGRAM

The average cost for medical assessment and treatment, psychological assessment and treatment, and physical therapy was $5,792 per patient. This figure is less than the previous average of $6,128.

CONCLUSIONS

1. Most patients rated their pain management program experience as very helpful.
2. Both immediately after the program and at follow-up, psychological treatments were rated more helpful than medical or physical therapy treatments.
3. Treatments that were rated most helpful at the end of the program were again rated most helpful 3 to 6 months after discharge.
4. Most patients reported improvements in activity and sleep at both discharge and follow-up.
5. Many patients referred to the Pain Management Program did not attain optimal expectancies.
6. A small minority of patients required hospitalizations and/or surgeries after discharge.

PLAN OF ACTION

1. Reassess individual outcome data to help identify those patients who are least likely to benefit from a structured outpatient pain program.

2. Incorporate an active vocational-rehabilitation component with functional capacity testing. Encourage greater incorporation of physical therapy into the program.
3. Scrutinize program goals of pain intensity, coping, and return to work.
4. Consider less intensive program in order to decrease costs.
5. Continue to collect and analyze outcome data.

SAMPLE HELPFULNESS QUESTIONNAIRE*

Pain Management Center
Brigham and Women's Hospital

❏ Posttreatment   Name: _____

❏ Follow-up   Date: _____

Below is a list of treatments offered at the Pain Management Center. Any treatment a person receives can be rated on a scale ranging from extremely harmful to extremely helpful, with neutral (not helpful or harmful) falling in the middle. If you had this treatment at *Brigham and Women's Hospital*, please rate it by making a vertical mark at the point on the line that indicates how helpful (or harmful) that treatment was to you. Leave blank any treatments you did not receive at Brigham and Women's Hospital.

	Extremely Harmful	*Harmful*	*Neutral*	*Helpful*	*Extremely Helpful*
Whole program					
Medical assessment and treatment					
Psychology assessment and treatment					
Physical therapy assessment and treatment					
Relaxation therapy					
Office visits with physician					
Individual physical therapy					
Individual psychological therapy					
Patient education groups					
Group therapy sessions					
Drug prescriptions					
Group exercise					
Individual exercise					
Trigger point nerve blocks					
Sympathetic nerve blocks					
Epidural steroid nerve blocks					
Biofeedback therapy (using biofeedback machine)					
Family conference sessions					

*Note. From *The Treatment Helpfulness Questionnaire: A Measure of Patient Satisfaction With Treatment Modalities Provided in Chronic Pain Management Programs*, by S. L. Chapman, R. N. Jamison, and S. H. Sanders, unpublished manuscript. Reprinted with permission.

Please answer the following brief questions:

1. Before I began the program at the Pain Management Center, my ability to cope with pain and related problems was

    ❏ Excellent   ❏ Good   ❏ Fair   ❏ Poor   ❏ Very poor

    a. I feel now that my ability to cope with pain and related problems is

    ❏ Excellent   ❏ Good   ❏ Fair   ❏ Poor   ❏ Very poor

2. Since the end of the program at the Pain Management Center, have you seen any health care professionals for the pain problem for which you were treated, aside from the routine follow-up visits?   ❏ Yes   ❏ No

    If no, skip to Question 3.

    a. On how many days did you visit a health care professional on an outpatient basis? _____ Please describe whom you saw and the treatment you received.

    b. Were you hospitalized because of your pain? ❏ Yes   ❏ No

        If so, please describe the reason and the treatment.

    c. Did you have surgery related to your pain? ❏ Yes   ❏ No

        If so, what kind of surgery?

3. Are you currently working for pay or involved daily in a vocational rehabilitation program?

    ❏ Yes   ❏ No

    If so, please indicate the nature of your job or program.

4. Complete this answer only if you had significant problems sleeping before beginning treatment at the Pain Management Center.

    Since treatment began, my ability to sleep is

    ❏ Significantly worse   ❏ Slightly worse   ❏ About the same   ❏ Slightly better   ❏ Significantly better

5. Do you think that plans for follow-up after the program were adequate? ❏ Yes   ❏ No

    If not, please explain.

6. Please rate your pain intensity on a scale from 0 = no pain to 10 = excruciating, incapacitating, worst pain possible. Write the *number* in the spaces below:

    a. Describes your pain at its worst   _____

    b. Describes your pain at its least   _____

    c. Describes your pain on the average _____

REFERENCES

Armentrout, D. P., Moore, J. E., Parker, J. C., Hewett, J. E., & Feltz, C. (1982). Pain patient MMPI subgroups: The psychological dimensions of pain. *Journal of Behavioral Medicine, 5,* 201-211.

Beck, A. T., & Steer, R. A. (1987). *Beck Depression Inventory Manual.* New York: Psychological Corporation.

Beck, A. T., Ward, C. H., Mendelson, M., Mock, J., & Erbaugh, J. (1961). An inventory for measuring depression. *Archives of General Psychiatry, 4,* 561-571.

Bergner, M., Bobbitt, R. A., Carter, W. B., & Gilson, B. S. (1981). The Sickness Impact Profile: Development and final revision of a health status measure. *Medical Care, 19,* 787-805.

Bonica, J. J. (1992). Preface. In G. Aronoff (Ed.), *Evaluation and Treatment of Chronic Pain* (2nd ed., p. xx.). Baltimore: Williams & Williams.

Bonica, J. J., & Loeser, J. D. (1990). Medical evaluation of the patient with pain. In J. J. Bonica (Ed.), *The Management of Pain* (Vol. 1, pp. 563-579). Philadelphia: Lea & Febiger.

Bradley, L. A., Prokop, C. K., Margolis, R., & Gentry, W. D. (1978). Multivariate analyses of the MMPI profiles of low back pain patients. *Journal of Behavioral Medicine, 1,* 253-272.

Brown, G. K., & Nicassio, P. M. (1987). The development of a questionnaire for the assessment of active and passive coping strategies in chronic pain patients. *Pain, 31,* 53-65.

Brown, G. K., Nicassio, P. M., & Wallston, K. A. (1989). Pain coping strategies and depression in rheumatoid arthritis. *Journal of Consulting and Clinical Psychology, 57,* 652-657.

Budzynski, T., Stoyva, J., Adler, L. S., & Mullaney, D. J. (1973). EMG biofeedback and tension headache: A controlled study. *Psychosomatic Medicine, 35,* 484-496.

Cairns, D., Mooney, V., & Crane, P. (1984). Spinal pain rehabilitation: Inpatient and outpatient treatment results and development of predictors for outcome. *Spine, 9,* 91.

Catalano, E. M. (Ed.). (1987). *The Chronic Pain Control Workbook: A Step-by-Step Guide for Coping With and Overcoming Your Pain.* Oakland, CA: New Harbinger.

Caudill, M., Schnable, R., Zuttermeister, P., Benson, H., & Friedman, R. (1991). Decreased clinic use by chronic pain patients: Response to behavioral medicine intervention. *The Clinical Journal of Pain, 7,* 305-310.

Chapman, S. L., Jamison, R. N., & Sanders, S. H. (unpublished manuscript). *The Treatment Helpfulness Questionnaire: A Measure of Patient Satisfaction With Treatment Modalities Provided in Chronic Pain Management Programs.*

Cinciripini, P. M., & Floreen, A. (1982). An evaluation of a behavioral program for chronic pain. *Journal of Behavioral Medicine, 5,* 375-389.

Commission on Accreditation of Rehabilitation Facilities. (1994). *Standards Manual for Organizations Serving People With Disabilities.* Tucson, AZ: Author.

Cousins, N. (1979). *Anatomy of an Illness as Perceived by the Patient.* New York: Bantam Books.

Davis, M., Eshelman, E. R., & McKay, M. (1982). *The Relaxation and Stress Reduction Workbook* (2nd ed.). Oakland, CA: New Harbinger.

Deardoff, W. W., Rubin, H. S., & Scott, D. W. (1991). Comprehensive multidisciplinary treatment of chronic pain: A follow-up study of treated and untreated groups. *Pain, 45,* 35-43.

DeGood, D. E., & Shutty, Jr., M. S. (1992). Assessment of pain beliefs, coping, and self-efficacy. In D. C. Turk & R. Melzack (Eds.), *Handbook of Pain Assessment* (pp. 214-234). New York: Guilford.

Derogatis, L. R. (1977). *The SCL-90-R: Administration, Scoring and Procedures Manual.* Baltimore: Clinical Psychometric Research.

Derogatis, L. R. (1983). *The SCL-90-R Manual II: Administration, Scoring and Procedures.* Towson, MD: Clinical Psychometric Research.

Egan, K. J. (1989). Behavioral analysis: The use of behavioral concepts to promote change of chronic pain patients. In J. D. Loeser & K. J. Egan (Eds.), *Managing the Chronic Pain Patient: Theory and Practice at the University of Washington Multidisciplinary Pain Center* (pp. 81-93). New York: Raven Press.

Erickson, R. K. (1989). The physical examination of the patient in pain. In P. M. Camic & F. D. Brown (Eds.), *Assessing Chronic Pain: A Multidisciplinary Clinic Handbook* (pp. 20-46). New York: Springer-Verlag.

Evans, J. H., & Kagan, A. (1986). The development of a functional rating scale to measure the treatment outcome of chronic spinal patients. *Spine, 11,* 277-281.

Ewings, J. A. (1984). Detecting alcoholism: The CAGE questionnaire. *Journal of the American Medical Association, 252,* 1905-1907.

Fairbank, J. C. T., Couper, J., Davies, J. B., & O'Brien, J. P. (1980). The Oswestry Low Back Pain Disability Questionnaire. *Physiotherapy, 66,* 271-273.

Flor, H., Fydrich, T., & Turk, D. C. (1992). Efficacy of multidisciplinary pain treatment centers: A meta-analytic review. *Pain, 49,* 221-230.

Flor, H., & Turk, D. C. (1984). Etiological theories and treatment for chronic back pain. I. Somatic models and interventions. *Pain, 19,* 105-121.

Follick, M. J., Ahern, D. K., & Aberger, E. W. (1987). Behavioral treatment of chronic pain. In J. A. Blumenthal & D. C. McKee (Eds.), *Applications in Behavioral Medicine and Health Psychology: A Clinician's Source Book* (pp. 237-270). Sarasota, FL: Professional Resource Exchange.

Follick, M. J., Ahern, D. K., & Laser-Wolston, N. (1984). Evaluation of a daily activity diary from chronic pain patients. *Pain, 19,* 373-382.

Follick, M. J., Smith, T. W., & Ahern, D. K. (1985). The Sickness Impact Profile: A global measure of disability in chronic low back pain. *Pain, 21,* 67-76.

Fordyce, W. E. (1976). *Behavioral Methods for Chronic Pain and Illness.* St. Louis: C. V. Mosby.

Frymoyer, J. W., & Cats-Baril, W. L. (1991). An overview of the incidence and costs of low back pain. *Orthopedics Clinics of North America, 22*(2), 263-271.

Gil, K., Williams, D. A., Keefe, F., & Beckham, J. C. (1990). The relationship of negative thoughts to pain and psychological distress. *Behavior Therapy, 21,* 349-362.

Hanson, R. W., & Gerber, K. W. (1990). *Coping With Chronic Pain: A Guide to Patient Self-Management.* New York: Guilford.

Hathaway, S. R., & McKinley, J. C. (1983). *Minnesota Multiphasic Personality Inventory: Manual for Administration and Scoring.* Minneapolis: University of Minnesota Press.

Hathaway, S. R., McKinley, J. C., Butcher, J. N., Dahlstrom, W. G., Graham, J. R., Tellegen, A., & Kaemmer, B. (1989). *Minnesota Multiphasic Personality Inventory-2: Manual for Administration.* Minneapolis: University of Minnesota Press.

Hilgard, A. D., & Hilgard, J. R. (1983). *Hypnosis in the Relief of Pain.* Los Altos, CA: William Kaufmann.

Holzman, A. D., & Turk, D. C. (Eds.). (1986). *Pain Management: A Handbook of Psychological Treatment Approaches.* New York: Pergamon.

Jamison, R. N. (1991). Psychological assessment of chronic pain. *Pain Digest, 1*, 230-237.

Jamison, R. N. (1996a). Comprehensive pretreatment and outcome assessment for chronic opioid therapy in nonmalignant pain. *Journal of Pain and Symptom Management, 11*, 231-241.

Jamison, R. N. (1996b). *Learning to Master Your Chronic Pain.* Sarasota, FL: Professional Resource Press.

Jamison, R. N., Anderson, K. O., Peeters-Asdourian, C., & Ferrante, F. M. (1994). Survey of opioid use in chronic nonmalignant pain patients. *Regional Anesthesia, 19*(4), 225-230.

Jamison, R. N., Rock, D. L., & Parris, W. C. V. (1988). Empirically derived Symptom Checklist 90 subgroups of chronic pain patients: A cluster analysis. *Journal of Behavioral Medicine, 11*, 147-158.

Jamison, R. N., Rudy, T. E., Penzien, D. B., & Mosley, T. H. (1994). Cognitive-behavioral classifications of chronic pain: Replication and extension of empirically derived patient profiles. *Pain, 57*, 277-292.

Jamison, R. N., Sbrocco, T., & Parris, W. C. V. (1989). The influence of physical and psychosocial factors on accuracy of memory for pain in chronic pain patients. *Pain, 37*, 289-294.

Jamison, R. N., Vasterling, J. J., & Parris, W. C. V. (1987). Use of sensory descriptors in assessing chronic pain patients. *Journal of Psychosomatic Research, 31*, 647-652.

Jamison, R. N., & Virts, K. L. (1990). The influence of family support on chronic pain. *Behavior Research and Therapy, 28*, 282-287.

Jensen, M. P., & Karoly, P. (1991). Control beliefs, coping efforts, and adjustment to chronic pain. *Journal of Consulting and Clinical Psychology, 59*, 431-438.

Jensen, M. P., Karoly, P., & Braver, S. (1986). The measurement of clinical pain intensity: A comparison of six methods. *Pain, 27*, 117-126.

Jensen, M. P., Karoly, P., & Huger, P. (1987). The development and preliminary validation of an instrument to assess patients' attitudes toward pain. *Journal of Psychosomatic Research, 31*, 393-400.

Jensen, M. P., & McFarland, C. A. (1993). Increasing the reliability and validity of pain intensity measurement in chronic pain patients. *Pain, 55*, 195-204.

Kames, L. D., Naliboff, B. D., Heinrich, R. L., & Schag, C. C. (1984). The Chronic Illness Problem Inventory: Problem-oriented psychosocial assessment of patients with chronic illness. *International Journal of Psychiatry in Medicine, 14*, 65-75.

Kaplan, R. M. (1993). Quality of life assessment for cost/utility studies in cancer. *Cancer Treatment Review, 19*(Suppl. 19), 85-96.

Keefe, F. S., & Block, A. R. (1982). Development of an observation method for assessing pain behavior in chronic low back pain patients. *Behavior Therapy, 13*, 363-375.

Kerns, R. D., Turk, D. C., & Rudy, T. E. (1985). The West Haven-Yale Multidimensional Pain Inventory. *Pain, 23,* 345-356.

Kubler-Ross, E. (1975). *On Death and Dying.* New York: Macmillan.

Leavitt, F. (1985). The value of MMPI conversion "V" in the assessment of psychogenic pain. *Journal of Psychosomatic Research, 29,* 125-131.

Lorig, K., Chastain, R. L., Ung, E., Shoor, S., & Holman, H. R. (1989). Development and evaluation of a scale to measure perceived self-efficacy in people with arthritis. *Arthritis and Rheumatism, 32,* 37-44.

Lynch, N. T., & Vasudevan, S. V. (Eds.). (1988). *Persistent Pain: Psychosocial Assessment and Intervention.* Boston: Kluwer Academic Publishers.

Maruta, T., Swanson, D. W., & McHardy, M. J. (1987). Three year follow-up of patients with chronic pain who were treated in a multidisciplinary pain management program. *Pain, 4*(Suppl. 4), 537.

Mayfield, D. G., McLeod, G., & Hall, P. (1984). The CAGE questionnaire: Validation of a new alcoholism screening instrument. *American Journal of Psychiatry, 131,* 1121-1123.

McCreary, C. (1985). Empirically derived MMPI profile clusters and characteristics of low back pain patients. *Journal of Consulting and Clinical Psychology, 53,* 558-560.

McKay, M., Davis, M., & Fanning, P. (1981). *Thoughts and Feelings: The Art of Cognitive Stress Interventions.* Oakland, CA: New Harbinger.

Melzack, R. (1975). The McGill Pain Questionnaire: Major properties and scoring methods. *Pain, 1,* 277-299.

Melzack, R. (1987). Short-Form McGill Pain Questionnaire. *Pain, 30,* 191-197.

Millon, T., Green, C. J., & Meagher, Jr., R. B. (1979). The MBHI: A new inventory for the psychodiagnostician in medical settings. *Professional Psychology, 10,* 529-539.

Moore, J. E., McCallum, S., Holman, C., & O'Brien, S. (1991, November). *Prediction of Return to Work After Pain Clinic Treatment by MMPI-2 Clusters.* Paper presented at the meeting of the American Pain Society, New Orleans, LA.

Moore, J. E., McFall, M. E., Kivlahan, D. R., & Capestany, F. (1988). Risk of misinterpretation of MMPI schizophrenia scale elevations in chronic pain patients. *Pain, 32,* 207-213.

Nepomeceno, C., Richards, J. S., & Urso, J. A. (1989). Accountability of pain control programs in the United States. *Southern Medical Journal, 82,* 1456.

Nicholas, M. K. (1992). Chronic pain. In P. H. Wilson (Ed.), *Principles and Practice of Relapse Prevention* (pp. 255-289). New York: Guilford.

Nigl, A. J. (1984). *Biofeedback and Behavioral Strategies in Pain Treatment.* Jamaica, NY: Spectrum Publications.

Nuprin Pain Report. (1985). New York: Louis Harris and Associates, Inc.

Parris, W. C. V., Jamison, R. N., & Vasterling, J. J. (1987). Follow-up study of a multidisciplinary pain center. *Journal of Pain and Symptom Management, 2*(2), 1-7.

Penzien, D. B., & Rains, J. C. (in press). *Self-Management Training Program for Chronic Headache: Patient Manual--Volume II.* Sarasota, FL: Professional Resource Press.

Pilowsky, I., & Spence, N. D. (1975). Patterns of illness behavior in patients with intractable pain. *Journal of Psychosomatic Research, 19,* 279-287.

Pilowsky, I., Spence, N. D., Cobb, J., & Katsikitis, M. (1984). The Illness Behavior Questionnaire as an aid to clinical assessment. *General Hospital Psychiatry, 6,* 123-130.

Pollard, C. A. (1984). Preliminary validity study of the Pain Disability Index. *Perception and Motor Skills, 59,* 974-984.

Portenoy, R. K. (1990). Chronic opioid therapy in nonmalignant pain. *Journal of Pain and Symptom Management, 5,* S46-S62.

Portenoy, R. K. (1994). Opioid therapy for chronic nonmalignant pain: Current status. In H. L. Fields & J. C. Liebeskind (Eds.), *Pharmacologic Approaches to the Treatment of Chronic Pain* (pp. 247-287). Seattle: IASP Publications.

Prokop, C. K., Bradley, L. A., Margolis, R., & Gentry, W. D. (1980). Multivariate analysis of the MMPI profiles of multiple pain patients. *Journal of Personality Assessment, 44,* 246-252.

Radloff, L. S. (1977). The Centers for Epidemiologic Studies-Depression Scale: A self-report depression scale for research in the general population. *Applied Psychological Measurement, 1,* 385-401.

Raj, P. P. (1992). History and physical examinations of the pain patient. In P. P. Raj (Ed.), *Practical Management of Pain* (2nd ed., pp. 81-121). St. Louis: Mosby - Year Book.

Roland, M., & Morris, R. (1983). A study of the natural history of back pain. Part I: Development of a reliable and sensitive measure of disability in low back pain. *Spine, 8,* 141-144.

Rosenstiel, A. K., & Keefe, F. J. (1983). The use of coping strategies in chronic low back pain patients: Relationship to patient characteristics and current adjustment. *Pain, 17,* 33-44.

Sanders, S. H. (1980). Toward a practical instrument system for the automatic measurement of "up-time" in chronic pain patients. *Pain, 9,* 103-109.

Savage, S. R. (1993). Addiction in the treatment of pain: Significance, recognition, and management. *Journal of Pain and Symptom Management, 8,* 265-278.

Schofferman, J. (1993). Long-term use of opioid analgesics for the treatment of chronic pain of nonmalignant origin. *Journal of Pain and Symptom Management, 8,* 279-288.

Schwartz, D. P. (1991). An algorithmic system for patient management in chronic pain programs. *Pain Digest, 1,* 183-190.

Seligman, M. E. P. (1994). *What You Can Change and What You Can't.* New York: Alfred A. Knopf.

Selye, H. (1956). *The Stress of Life.* New York: McGraw-Hill.

Selye, H. (1975). *From Dream to Discovery.* Montreal, Canada: International Institute of Stress.

Selzer, M. L. (1971). The Michigan alcoholism screening test: The quest for a new diagnostic instrument. *American Journal of Psychiatry, 127,* 275-286.

Steedman, S. M., Middaugh, S. J., Kee, W. G., Carson, D. S., Harden, R. N., & Miller, M. C. (1992). Chronic pain medications: Equivalence levels and method of quantifying usage. *The Clinical Journal of Pain, 8,* 204-214.

Swenson, W. M., & Morse, R. M. (1975). The use of a self-administered alcoholism screen test (SAAST) in a medical center. *Mayo Clinic Proceedings, 50,* 204-208.

Tollison, C. D., Kriegl, M. L., & Downie, G. R. (1985). Chronic low back pain: Results of treatment at the Pain Therapy Center. *Southern Medical Journal, 78,* 1291.

Turk, D. C., & Flor, H. (1984). Etiological theories and treatments from chronic back pain. II. Psychological models and interventions. *Pain, 19,* 209-233.

Turk, D. C., & Melzack, R. (1992). The measurement of pain and the assessment of people experiencing pain. In D. C. Turk & R. Melzack (Eds.), *Handbook of Pain Assessment* (pp. 3-12). New York: Guilford.

Turk, D. C., & Rudy, T. E. (1988). Toward an empirically-derived taxonomy of chronic pain patients: Integration of psychological assessment data. *Journal of Consulting and Clinical Psychology, 56,* 233-238.

Vasudevan, S. V. (1992). Impairement, disability, and functional capacity assessment. In D. C. Turk & R. Melzack (Eds.), *Handbook of Pain Assessment* (pp. 100-108). New York: Guilford.

Waddell, G. (1982). An approach to backache. *British Journal of Hospital Medicine, 28,* 187-219.

Waddell, G., & Main, C. J. (1984). Assessment of severity in low back disorders. *Spine, 9,* 204-208.

Ware, J. E., & Sherbourne, C. D. (1992). The MOS 36-item Short-Form Health Survey (SF-36). *Medical Care, 30,* 473-483.

Williams, J. B., Gibbon, M., First, M. B., Spitzer, R. L., Davis, M., Borus, J., Howes, M. J., Kane, J., Pope, H. G., Rounsaville, B., & Wittchen, H. U. (1992). The structured clinical interview for *DSM-III-R. Archives of General Psychiatry,* 49, 630-636.

World Health Organization. (1986). *Cancer Pain Relief.* Geneva: Author.

ADDITIONAL RESOURCES

FOR CHAPTER 1 -
THEORETICAL ISSUES OF CHRONIC PAIN

Elton, D., Stanley, G., & Burrows, G. (1983). *Psychological Control of Pain*. Sidney, Australia: Grune & Stratton.

This book is useful for a review of theoretical and methodological issues of pain. Psychological and medical approaches to pain are discussed.

Turk, D. C., Meichenbaum, D., & Genest, M. (1983). *Pain and Behavioral Medicine: A Cognitive-Behavioral Perspective*. New York: Guilford.

This book reviews psychologically oriented approaches and cognitive-behavioral techniques in the treatment of chronic pain.

Wall, P. D., & Jones, M. (1991). *Defeating Pain: The War Against A Silent Epidemic*. New York: Plenum.

This book provides an easy-to-understand explanation of the causes and mechanisms of pain and explores the different ways people have learned to deal with pain.

FOR CHAPTER 2 -
PROGRAM DESCRIPTION

Blumenthal, J. A., & McKee, D. C. (Eds.).   (1987).   *Applications in Behavioral Medicine and Health Psychology: A Clinician's Source Book.*   Sarasota, FL: Professional Resource Exchange.

Two chapters should be consulted in this text: "Observational Methods for Assessing Pain: A Practical Guide" by Francis Keefe, James Crisson, and Mary Trainor, and "Behavioral Treatment of Chronic Pain" by Michael Follick, David Ahern, and Edward Aberger.

Hanson, R. W., & Gerber, K. E. (1990).   *Coping With Chronic Pain: A Guide To Patient Self-Management.* New York: Guilford.

This is a book for the practicing clinician on the biopsychosocial perspective of assessment and treatment of chronic pain. There is a very useful chapter on the organization and management of a chronic pain program.

Loeser, J. D., & Egan, K. J. (Eds.). (1989).   *Managing the Chronic Pain Patient: Theory and Practice at the University of Washington Multidisciplinary Pain Center.* New York: Raven Press.

A multiauthored book on programmatic issues in the management of chronic pain. The book contains useful chapters on cognitive-behavioral therapy, vocational issues for chronic pain patients, and the organization of an inpatient pain treatment program.

Philips, H. C. (1988).   *The Psychological Management of Chronic Pain: A Treatment Manual.* New York: Springer.

This is a practical guide on treatment strategies and instructional information used in a pain management program.

FOR CHAPTER 3 -
ASSESSMENT AND
PATIENT SELECTION ISSUES

Camic, P. M., & Brown, F. D. (Eds.). (1989). *Assessing Chronic Pain: A Multidisciplinary Handbook.* New York: Springer-Verlag.

Each chapter in this text is authored by a member of a different discipline involved in a multidisciplinary pain clinic.

Karoly, P., & Jensen, M. P. (1987). *Multimethod Assessment of Chronic Pain.* New York: Pergamon.

This book reviews the various methods used for pain assessment. Critical appraisals of each assessment technique are particularly helpful.

Turk, D. C., & Melzack, R. (Eds.). (1992). *Handbook of Pain Assessment.* New York: Guilford.

This comprehensive text includes reviews of medical and psychological evaluation techniques of patients with pain. Attention to specialty topics is especially valuable.

Wall, P. D., & Melzack, R. (Eds.). (1994). *Textbook of Pain* (3rd ed.). New York: Churchill Livingstone.

This is an authoritative, comprehensive volume composed of 81 chapters by 125 authors covering all aspects of pain from basic science to clinical intervention.

FOR CHAPTER 4 -
DIDACTIC SESSIONS

Davis, M., Eshelman, E. R., & McKay, M. (1982). *The Relaxation and Stress Reduction Workbook* (2nd ed.). Oakland, CA: New Harbinger.

This workbook was written for the general public with specific exercises to reduce stress. This volume has many practical resources and valuable techniques.

Linden, W. (1990). *Autogenic Training: A Clinical Guide.* New York: Guilford.

A thorough introduction to autogenic relaxation.

Lynch, N. T., & Vasudevan, S. V. (Eds.). (1988). *Persistent Pain: Psychosocial Assessment and Intervention.* Boston: Kluwer Academic Publishers.

This is a comprehensive text that has valuable chapters on behavioral assessment, vocational rehabilitation, and disability issues.

Nigl, A. J. (1984). *Biofeedback and Behavioral Strategies in Pain Treatment.* New York: Spectrum Publications.

This is a useful text on the overview of biofeedback techniques and relaxation strategies.

Wilson, P. H. (Ed.). (1992). *Principles and Practice of Relapse Prevention.* New York: Guilford.

Each chapter in this book reviews relapse prevention strategies for a particular disorder. Most useful is a chapter on relapse prevention for treatment of chronic pain.

FOR CHAPTER 5 - THERAPY ISSUES

Cowles, J. (1993). *Pain Relief! How to Say "No" to Acute, Chronic, and Cancer Pain.* New York: Mastermedia Limited.

This is a comprehensive book on the assessment and treatment of pain which was written for the general public. It contains many helpful resources.

Lang, S. S., & Patt, R. B. (1994). *You Don't Have To Suffer: A Complete Guide to Relieving Cancer Pain for Patients and Their Families.* New York: Oxford University Press.

An excellent guide for treating and dealing with cancer pain. This book is a useful source for information on medication used in treating pain.

Roy, R. (1989). *Chronic Pain and the Family: A Problem-Centered Perspective.* New York: Human Sciences Press.

This book explores the consequences of chronic pain on marital relationships and family functioning. It includes many case reports.

Tunks, E., & Bellissimo, A. (1991). *Behavioral Medicine: Concepts and Procedures.* Elmsford, NY: Pergamon.

This book provides reliable information about the etiology of common disorders and contains practical guidelines for treatment.

Woolfolk, R. L., & Lehrer, P. M. (1984). *Principles and Practice of Stress Management.* New York: Guilford.

This is an edited book of relaxation and stress reduction techniques for the practitioner.

Yost, E. B., & Corbishley, M. A. (1987). *Career Counseling: A Psychological Approach*. San Francisco: Jossey-Bass.

This book gives a step-by-step approach to provide career counseling to patients which integrates psychological and vocational assessment and intervention techniques.

FOR CHAPTER 6 -
PROGRAM EVALUATION

Commission on Accreditation of Rehabilitation Facilities. (1987). *Program Evaluation in Chronic Pain Management Programs*. Tucson, AZ: Author.

This guide was produced to help guide members of a chronic pain management center develop a market-driven evaluation system.

Commission on Accreditation of Rehabilitation Facilities. (1993). *Standards Manual for Organizations Serving People With Disabilities*. Tucson, AZ: Author.

This guide presents standards for an accredited pain management center.

Davis, J. B. (1991). *365 Ways to Manage the Business Called Private Practice: Practical Management Techniques That You Can Use Today to Improve the Success of Your Medical Practice*. Los Angeles: Practice Management Information Corporation.

This easy-to-read book contains a variety of ideas proven to be effective in improving business practices.

HealthCare Consultants of America, Inc. (1993). *Business Aspects of Medical Practice: Strategies to Ensure Success in Today's Rapidly Changing Medical Practice Environment*. Augusta, GA: Author.

This handbook contains information for practice managers and administrators on setting up, organizing, and marketing a medical practice. Useful information is given on managed care and billing issues.

McCue, J. D., & Ficalora, R. D. (1991). *Private Practice: A Guide to Getting Started*. Boston: Little, Brown and Company.

This is a practitioners "how-to" book on improving practice management and making effective business decisions.

APPENDIX:
COMMONLY PRESCRIBED MEDICATIONS

COMMONLY USED
NONPRESCRIPTION ANALGESICS

Generic Name	Brand Name (Examples)	Standard Dose*	Comments
Aspirin	Bufferin, Anacin, Excedrin	650 to 1,000 mg	• Used as standard of comparison • May irritate the stomach, cause gastrointestinal bleeding; increases platelet bleeding time • Commercial products may also include caffeine and other additives
Acetaminophen	Tylenol, Panadol, Anacin-3, Tempra, Datril	650 to 1,000 mg	• Similar to aspirin in analgesic effects but no anti-inflammatory effects • Doesn't irritate the stomach • May cause liver damage in very high doses
Ibuprofen	Advil, Nuprin, Motrin, Ibuprin, Midol 200, Dolgesic, Pamprin	400 to 800 mg	• Possible side effects include renal and cardiovascular problems, ringing in the ears, gastrointestinal upset, kidney and liver problems

*All medication taken orally unless otherwise indicated.

COMMONLY USED NONSTEROIDAL
ANTI-INFLAMMATORY DRUGS (NSAIDS)

Generic Name	Brand Name	Standard Dose*	Comments
Choline magnesium trisalicylate	Trilisate	1,000 to 1,500 mg	• Pill or liquid form • Recommended when there is a history of gastric bleeding
Diclofenac	Voltaren	50 to 75 mg	• Coated to reduce stomach upset • Comparable in safety to ibuprofen and naproxen • High doses may cause liver toxicity
Diflunisal	Dolobid	500 to 1,000 mg	• Lasts longer than aspirin or ibuprofen • Usually taken twice a day • Less irritating to stomach than aspirin
Etodolac	Lodine	200 to 400 mg	• Causes less gastrointestinal bleeding than other NSAIDS
Fenoprofen	Nalfon	200 to 600 mg	• Comparable to aspirin; may cause renal problems • Short-acting
Flurbiprofen	Ansaid	50 to 100 mg	• Longer duration of action (6 to 8 hours) • Doses limited to 300 mg per day
Indomethacin	Indocin	25 to 50 mg	• High incidence of adverse effects, including drowsiness; may cause renal problems • Available as rectal suppository

*All medication taken orally unless otherwise indicated.

Generic Name	Brand Name	Standard Dose	Comments
Ketoprofen	Orudis	25 to 75 mg	• Comparable to 400 mg of ibuprofen and superior to 650 mg of aspirin • Rapid onset; long duration of action
Ketorolac	Toradol	30 to 60 mg (injectable); 10 mg	• If injected, use should be limited to 5 days • Oral dose indicated only as continuation therapy to injectable; not to exceed 5 days
Meclofenamate	Meclomen, Meclofen	50 to 100 mg	• Comparable to aspirin • Duration of 4 to 8 hours • May cause diarrhea; less risk of stomach upset
Nabumetone	Relafen	1,000 to 2,000 mg	• May take 1 to 2 weeks to reach maximal effectiveness
Naproxen	Naprosyn	250 to 500 mg	• Slower onset and longer duration of action (8 to 12 hours)
Naproxen sodium	Anaprox	275 to 550 mg	• Similar to naproxen
Piroxicam	Feldene	20 mg	• Taken once a day • Good for patients who do not comply with multiple doses
Sulindac	Clinoril, Arthorobid	150 to 200 mg	• Not as problematic with regard to kidney function as indomethacin
Tolmetin	Tolectin	400 mg	• Weak analgesic effect • Short half-life (60 minutes)

COMMONLY USED
OPIOID ANALGESICS

Generic Name	Brand Name	Standard Dose*	Comments
Butorphanol	Stadol, Stadol NS	0.5 to 1.0 mg (injectable)	• Comes in nasal spray that is equivalent to injection
Codeine	Codeine (often combined with other products, e.g., Tylenol #3, Empirin)	30 to 60 mg	• Usually combined with aspirin or acetaminophen
Fentanyl	Sublimaze, Dura-gesic	0.1 mg (injectable); 25 g/hr (patch)	• Short-acting when injected • Long-acting as a transdermal patch (> 72 hours); withdrawal symptoms possible after patch removal
Hydrocodone	Vicodin, Lortab, Hycodan, Hydro-cet, Bancap	5 mg	• 10 mg equivalent to 90 mg of codeine • Often combined with aspirin or acetaminophen
Hydromorphone	Dilaudid	4 to 8 mg; 1.3 mg (injectable)	• Available as high potency injectable preparation and as suppository
Oxycodone	Percodan, Perco-cet, Roxicet, Ty-lox, Roxicodone	5 mg	• 10 mg equivalent to 90 mg of codeine • Most often combined with acetaminophen or aspirin; toxicity possible with higher doses

*All medication taken orally unless otherwise indicated.

Generic Name	Brand Name	Standard Dose	Comments
Oxycodone; controlled release	Oxycontin	10 mg	• 8 to 12 hour sustained-release tablets
Meperidine	Demerol	50 to 400 mg; 50 to 100 mg (injectable)	• Potential for excitability and convulsions • Injectable dose lasts between 2 to 4 hours • Not recommended for chronic use
Methadone	Dolophine	10 to 20 mg; 10 mg (injectable)	• Long-acting opioid • Good analgesia without euphoria
Morphine	Roxanol, MSIR, Duramorph	5 to 30 mg 2 to 10 mg (injectable)	• Standard to which other opioids are compared
Morphine; controlled-release	Oramorph SR, MS Contin	30 to 100 mg	• 8- to 12-hour sustained-release tablets
Oxymorphone	Numorphan	1.1 mg (injectable)	• Injectable dose lasts 3 to 5 hours • Available as suppository
Pentazocine	Talwin	50 mg; 60 mg (injectable)	• Injectable dose lasts 2 to 4 hours • Oral dose equivalent to codeine
Propoxyphene	Darvon, Darvocet, Wygesic	65 mg	• Combined with aspirin or aceta-minophen • May cause dysphoria and hallucinations
Tramadol	Ultram	50 mg	• As effective as morphine with low abuse potential

COMMONLY USED
ANTIDEPRESSANTS

Generic Name	Brand Name	Standard Dose*	Comments
Amitriptyline	Elavil	10 to 25 mg	• Frequently prescribed for chronic pain patients • Can sedate and aid sleep • Helps to improve mood • May cause dry mouth, drowsiness, and weight gain
Amoxapine	Asendin	200 to 300 mg	• Occasionally associated with sudden involuntary movements (e.g., jerking)
Desipramine	Norpramine	75 to 300 mg	• Fewer adverse effects than other tricyclic antidepressants
Doxepin	Sinequan	75 to 300 mg	• Similar to amitriptyline
Fluoxetine	Prozac	20 to 80 mg	• May produce nervousness, insomnia, and weight loss • Fewer adverse effects than other tricyclic antide-pressants • Single daily dose • Efficacy for pain unproven
Imipramine	Tofranil	20 to 300 mg	• Less sedating than amitriptyline

*All medication taken orally unless otherwise indicated.

Generic Name	Brand Name	Standard Dose	Comments
Maprotiline	Ludiomil	75 to 300 mg	• Sedating with few other adverse effects
Nortriptyline	Pamelor, Aventyl	50 to 100 mg	• Lower incidences of adverse effects than with amitriptyline • Used with cardiac patients
Paroxetine	Paxil	20 to 50 mg	• Similar to sertraline and fluoxetine; may cause restlessness
Sertraline	Zoloft	50 to 200 mg	• May cause gastrointestinal symptoms, tremor, mania, insomnia, and sexual dysfunction
Trazodone	Desyrel	150 to 400 mg	• May cause inappropriate erections in males

COMMONLY USED MINOR
TRANQUILIZERS AND MUSCLE RELAXANTS

Generic Name	Brand Name	Standard Dose*	Comments
Alprazolam	Xanax	0.25 to 1 mg	• Antianxiety medication; dependence and withdrawal reactions with seizures possible
Baclofen	Lioresil	10 to 50 mg	• Muscle relaxant
Carisoprodol	Soma	350 to 700 mg	• Muscle relaxant
Chloroxazone	Parafon Forte	500 to 750 mg	• Muscle relaxant; minimal adverse effect reported
Clonazepam	Klonopin	0.5 to 2 mg	• Anticonvulsant • Useful for nerve pain • Extreme drowsiness and weakness possible
Clorazepate	Tranxene	15 to 60 mg	• Dizziness and gastrointestinal symptoms possible
Cyclobenzaprine	Flexeril	20 to 30 mg	• Muscle relaxant
Diazepam	Valium	5 to 10 mg	• Helpful in reducing anxiety • May cause depression • Not to be combined with alcohol • Not helpful for chronic anxiety; may cause dependency
Lorazepam	Ativan	1 to 5 mg	• Antianxiety and sedating effects • May produce physical dependence
Methocarbamol	Robaxin	500 to 1,000 mg; 10 ml (injectable)	• Muscle relaxant; oral and injectable

*All medication taken orally unless otherwise indicated.

Generic Name	Brand Name	Standard Dose	Comments
Temazepam	Restoril	15 to 30 mg	• Only for short-term insomnia; dizziness and light headedness possible
Triazolam	Halcion	0.125 to 0.50 mg	• Only for short-term insomnia • Risk of memory problems, tolerance, and dependence

COMMONLY PRESCRIBED ANTICONVULSANT MEDICATIONS

Generic Name	Brand Name	Standard Dose*	Comments
Carbamazepine	Tegretol	100 to 500 mg	• Adverse effects include dizziness, loss of coordination, sedation, confusion, liver and bone marrow damage • Blood levels should be periodically monitored • Liquid form available
Clonazepam	Klonopin, Rivotril	0.5 to 2 mg	• Dizziness, sedation, and fatigue are common
Phenytoin	Dilantin, Epanutine	100 to 300 mg	• May affect gum tissue in mouth; regular dental hygiene needed • Other adverse effects include acne, hair growth, liver and bone marrow damage
Valproic acid	Depakene	250 to 500 mg	• Adverse effects include pancreatitis, nausea, insomnia, headache, liver damage, and tremor

*All medication taken orally unless otherwise indicated.

SUBJECT INDEX

A

Acute Pain, 3
American Pain Society, 2
Anxiety, 2
Assertiveness Training, 86, 88, 89

B

Behavioral Analysis, 23
Behavioral Model, 5
Biofeedback, 11, 12, 69
Biomedical Model, 5
Biopsychosocial Model, 5

C

Chronic Pain, 3, 4
Cognitive/Behavioral Therapy, 56, 57
Comfort Measures, 86
Compliance, 61
Comprehensive Pain Questionnaire, 35-43
Computed Tomography (CT), 15
Concentration, 97

N

Negative Thinking, 89, 90
Neuropathic Pain, 16
Neurosurgical Treatments, 88
Numerical Pain Ratings, 20, 39, 137
Nuprin Pain Report, 3
Nutrition, 12, 93, 94

O

Occupational Therapy, 12
Opioid Therapy Contract, 107
Opioids, 79, 80
Organic Pain, 4, 5

P

Pain, 3, 4
       Acute, 3
       Chronic, 3, 4
Pain Intensity, 18-20
       Numerical Rating Scales, 19, 20
       Pain Drawings, 19
       Verbal Rating Scales, 19-21
       Visual Analogue Scales, 19
Pain Treatments
       Acupuncture, 6, 12, 87
       Implantable Devices, 88
       Injections, Nerve Blocks, 6, 12, 87
       Magnotherapy, 87
       Manipulation, 6
       Massage, 87
       Medication, 78-82, 87
       Psychotherapy, 6, 12
       Transcutaneous Electrical Nerve Stimulation, 6, 12, 87
Pathology, 16
Patient Contract, 13-14
Patient Education, 67-68
Patient Rating System, 59-61

MULTIMEDIA VERSION OF
LEARNING TO MASTER YOUR CHRONIC PAIN

Computer-assisted instructional software is being developed to accompany the *Learning to Master Your Chronic Pain* handbook. CD-ROM software will be available in both Microsoft Windows and Macintosh versions.

This software will offer a number of unique features including:

- "Live" relaxation sessions including your choice of sessions which include (a) diaphragmatic breathing, (b) progressive muscle relaxation, (c) autogenic relaxation, and (d) imagery

- Timed stretching exercises that can be customized for your specific pain problem

- Your choice of background sounds (music and/or voice-over instructions)

- Features to enhance your learning including quizzes, checklists, interactive exercises, multiple choice reviews, a glossary of terms, and cross-referencing

- Procedures for recording your pain, mood, activity, medication use, and personal comments plus information on your individual progress that can be stored, analyzed, and printed out for your use or for use by a healthcare professional

In order to use this software, you will need the following minimum computer system:

Windows Version: IBM-compatible PC with an 80486 or higher processor; Windows 3.1 or higher operating system; a hard disk with at least 8 MB of free space; a CD-ROM drive (minimum 2X speed, faster speed preferred); 4MB of available RAM (8MB preferred for Windows 95); sound card and speakers; a mouse; SVGA monitor with graphics adapter; and printer with graphics capabilities.

Macintosh Version: Macintosh computer with 68030 or higher processor; Version 6 or higher operating system; a hard disk with at least 8 MB of free space; a CD-ROM drive (minimum 2X speed, faster speed preferred); 4MB of available RAM; a mouse; 640 X 480 screen with 256 colors; and printer with graphics capabilities.

If you would like to receive more information when this CD-ROM Pain Management Program becomes available, please complete and return this form:

Name (Please Print All Info):_____

Address:_____

Address:_____

City:_____ State: _____ Zip:_____

Profession:_____

Write: Professional Resource Press, PO Box 15560, Sarasota, FL 34277-1560
Phone: 941-366-7913   **FAX:** 941-366-7971   **E-mail:** prpress@aol.com

If You Found This Book Useful . . .

You might want to know more about our other titles.

If you would like to receive our latest catalog, please return this form.

Name: _____
(Please Print)

Address: _____

Address: _____

City/State/Zip: _____

I am a:

❐ Psychologist   ❐ Mental Health Counselor
❐ Physician   ❐ Marriage and Family Therapist
❐ Clinical Social Worker   ❐ School Psychologist
❐ Nurse   ❐ Other: _____
❐ Psychiatrist

Write: Professional Resource Press, P.O. Box 15560, Sarasota, FL 34277-1560
Phone: 941-366-7913   **FAX:** 941-366-7971   **E-mail:** prpress@aol.com

MCP/7/96

- -

Add A Colleague To Our Mailing List . . .

If you would like us to send our latest catalog to one of your colleagues, please return this form.

Name: _____
(Please Print)

Address: _____

Address: _____

City/State/Zip: _____

This person is a:

❐ Psychologist   ❐ Mental Health Counselor
❐ Physician   ❐ Marriage and Family Therapist
❐ Clinical Social Worker   ❐ School Psychologist
❐ Nurse   ❐ Other: _____
❐ Psychiatrist

Write: Professional Resource Press, P.O. Box 15560, Sarasota, FL 34277-1560
Phone: 941-366-7913   **FAX:** 941-366-7971   **E-mail:** prpress@aol.com

MCP/7/96